REFLEX ACTIVITY OF
THE SPINAL CORD

REFLEX ACTIVITY
OF THE
SPINAL CORD

BY

R. S. CREED, D. DENNY-BROWN
J. C. ECCLES, E. G. T. LIDDELL
AND C. S. SHERRINGTON

REPRINTED

WITH ANNOTATIONS BY

D. P. C. LLOYD

Professor
Rockefeller University, New York
Honorary Research Fellow of
University College, London

OXFORD
AT THE CLARENDON PRESS

Oxford University Press, Ely House, London W. 1

GLASGOW NEW YORK TORONTO MELBOURNE WELLINGTON
CAPE TOWN IBADAN NAIROBI DAR ES SALAAM LUSAKA ADDIS ABABA
DELHI BOMBAY CALCUTTA MADRAS KARACHI LAHORE DACCA
KUALA LUMPUR SINGAPORE HONG KONG TOKYO

FIRST PRINTED 1932
REPRINTED 1972

*Printed in Great Britain
at the University Press, Oxford
by Vivian Ridler
Printer to the University*

PREFACE TO THE ORIGINAL EDITION

THIS small book attempts on behalf of the student of medicine —indeed on behalf of any student interested in the physiology of the nervous system—a concise account of elementary features of reflex mechanism, as illustrated particularly by the mammalian spinal cord.

To that end the plan here followed is to introduce and describe *seriatim* a number of reflexes typically obtainable from the mammalian preparation. These in every instance are reflexes which take expression in the skeletal musculature, predominantly in that of the limbs. The description and discussion given of them in each case are directed mainly towards analysis of the working of the reflex mechanism. In that connexion an object of study kept in view throughout is the individual motor-unit as a basal element of the reflex response. Improved technique provides more precise observations than were formerly possible of reflex time-relations and reflex quantities of effect both mechanical and electrical; hence the interpretation of reflex response in terms of the motor-unit itself becomes a tangible objective.

The anatomical range of the book extends no farther headward than the quadrigeminal region of the brain. The higher actions of the nervous system are of set purpose omitted. The scope of the book extends to reflexes within the strict meaning of that term. Its discussion of them comprises finally an attempt to trace general principles of co-ordination observable in them, and in their interaction.

The theme of the book being reflex mechanism it undertakes no systematic review of reflexes from their aspect as items of animal 'behaviour' or 'conduct'. In short, of questions raised by reflex action, with all its variety of 'reflex figure' and 'pattern', the problem dealt with here is that of physiological production and execution, and not that of biological significance.

In the bibliography appended we have had in mind especially the convenience of students who are accustomed to consult works written in English. The list selected does not pretend to completeness.

vi PREFACE

Lastly we would add that although our pages make little explicit reference to clinical fact and study, we yet cherish the hope that the student may find in them matter helpful to him when, under the guidance of his clinical teachers, he encounters the problems of nervous action presented in neurological practice.

R. S. C.
D. D.-B.
J. C. E.
E. G. T. L.
C. S. S.

The thanks of his fellow collaborators are gratefully given to their colleague, E. G. T. L., for his care, at the cost of much time and trouble, in assembling and adjusting contributions written somewhat individually for final incorporation in the text.

PREFACE TO THE 1972 REPRINT

THIS book is of much more than historical interest. It is a condensation of existing knowledge at the time of its first publication. It is a lineal descendent from Sherrington's *Integrative action of the nervous system*. The *Integrative action* was reprinted in 1947 on the occasion of the International Physiological Congress meeting in Oxford. This book is worthy of comparable treatment. It presents the elements that the student and experimenter utilizing the most modern instruments yet should have at hand if he is to make some sense of his efforts in terms of the whole organism.

This attempt at annotation for a second edition of the *Reflex activity of the spinal cord* has been a rewarding and worthwhile venture, although more difficult in its execution than had been imagined at the outset—rewarding and worth-while because of its great intrinsic value and because of its unavailability to students of the spinal cord and indeed to neurologists and neurophysiologists generally.

An early decision was to preserve the text unchanged. Hence the use of appended amendments or annotations in this edition. Their purpose essentially is to bridge the gap between primary use of the myograph and primary use of the direct coupled amplifier *cum* cathode-ray oscilloscope for analysis of spinal reflex activity, a gradual change spread over perhaps a decade but nevertheless one that coincided generally with the publication of this book. They do not pretend to present the latest word. Their scope is, in a word, limited.

At the time this book was published the flexor reflex was considered to be the simplest reflex reaction. With the advent of satisfactory oscillography substituting direct recording from nerves and central neurones for the indirect indications yielded by muscle action this was found not to be so. More accurate measures of nerve conduction velocity were made. After-potentials were proved to be real and normal events whereas previously they had been suspect. A consideration of them today is vital to any interpretation of elementary central action. The monosynaptic reflex as an unique entity linking primary afferent fibres directly with motoneurones was established, proving finally and incidentally to represent, as it were, a fractional form of the stretch reflex. Flexor reflexes were found to contain interneurones in their minimum pathway and so could no longer be employed to test events at the motoneurone. Monosynaptic reflexes took their place, by the use of which advances in the understanding of excitatory and inhibitory states in the spinal cord were made.

Inevitably the language of neurophysiology has changed— another reason for the addition of notes rather than alteration of the text. All those who have urged reissue have desired retention of the original text. As the purpose is to bring this book into currency this has been done. Despite advances it contains the foundation for present-day work and thought. In the question of added references there exist suitable monographs that will convey the information contained in a number of original papers. When it has been possible, for everyone's convenience, reference has been made to them.

1971   D. P. C. L.

FOREWORD

By E. G. T. LIDDELL

IN 1932, when this book first appeared, mechanical devices for analysis in neuro-muscular physiology were giving way to electrical methods. In its time, however, the mechanical myograph had been extremely valuable, especially in the hands of Sherrington.

In 1899 he had delivered his Marshall Hall address 'On the spinal animal'. Encouraged by W. H. Gaskell, he had explored the actions of muscles controlled by the spinal centres, after the cord had been isolated from higher centres, and so not under their control (cf. François-Franck, 1887, *Fonctions motrices du Cerveau*). Sherrington found that antagonistic muscles of limbs do not co-operate in the sense that they 'contract synchronously with the prime muscle as Winslow and Ducherre had supposed. Instead, they are inhibited. This discovery was the basis of his subsequent work. 'For instance', he wrote, 'when the motor nerves of the flexor muscles are excited, the motor nerves of the extensor muscles are simultaneously inhibited.'

In 1932, after 30 industrious years, Sherrington, with some of his pupils, reviewed their field of neurophysiology and put together a number of essays under the title *Reflex activity of the spinal cord*. Now, after some 40 years, when the old book is only a record of times past but nevertheless in some demand, it has seemed to D. P. C. Lloyd and A. K. McIntyre that it should be reprinted, but modified and modernized so as to link the old with the new. Hence comes this new edition.

ACKNOWLEDGEMENTS

IT is a pleasure to take this opportunity of acknowledging our indebtedness for help to several friends and colleagues: to Professor Adrian with his collaborators Dr. Zotterman and Professor Bronk for illustrations from their published papers; to Mr. B. H. C. Matthews for use of his original record, our figure 23; to Mr. E. C. Hoff for the microphotographs furnishing figure 5.

Sir Edward Sharpey Schafer has kindly allowed us to reproduce the text figure from *Essentials of Histology* (Edition 1929, Sir Edward Sharpey Schafer with the co-operation of H. M. Carleton).

We also thank the Royal Society for the electrotypes of figures 46, 53*b*, and for the facility of reproducing a number of other figures from the Society's Proceedings B., and also the *Journal of Physiology* for similar permission. To all these we extend our hearty thanks.

ACKNOWLEDGEMENTS TO THE
1972 REPRINT

I THANK the following for permission to use illustrations in these addenda: the American Physiological Society for figures from the *Handbook of Physiology*, *Sec. 1, Vol. 2, 1960*, and from the *Journal of Neurophysiology*; the Otago Medical School Research Society *Proceedings*, Dunedin, N.Z.; the Rockefeller University Press for figures originally published in the *Journal of General Physiology*; and the National Academy of Sciences (U.S.A.) for an illustration from its *Proceedings*.

I am grateful to Professor E. G. T. Liddell for reviewing these addenda and to Professor D. E. Denny-Brown who has contributed a beautifully executed modernized version of the original Fig. 71. Professor A. K. McIntyre of Monash University, Clayton, Victoria, Australia, has played an important part in this effort.

Finally, I thank Professor J. Z. Young and Professor P. D. Wall for their kind provision of facilities at University College London which have made these annotations possible.

D. P. C. L.

CONTENTS

FIGS. 2; 3–4; 5 *a*, *b*; 22–24; 25, 27, 30; 44; 46; 53 *a*, *b* and 67;
69 *a*, *b*; 71; are contained in separate plates facing pp. 2, 3, 5,
56, 57, 85, 89, 99, 162, 166.

I

THE REFLEX ARC

[168, 96]

IF a piece of blotting-paper is moistened with weak acid and laid upon the skin of a decapitated frog, it excites a train of movements by which the animal gets rid of the irritating agent. The movements are reflex. The response involves a chain of reactions, which, starting in the skin, travel by the nerves from the skin to the spinal cord and thence back to the periphery to the muscles which, in the example cited, are conveniently termed 'effector organs'. After the spinal cord is destroyed, no action is evoked. Cutting the nerve between the skin and the spinal cord will also abolish the reflex. Similarly, severance of the nerve from the spinal cord to the muscles precludes any reflex movement. In such types of reflex response the path travelled is a simple 'reflex arc' (Fig. 1), and consists of

(a) The inward path, which is composed of a receptor organ connected to an afferent nerve-fibre. Afferent nerve-fibres enter the spinal cord by the dorsal roots.

(b) The nervous (or reflex) centre in the central nervous system.

(c) The outward path, composed of an efferent nerve-fibre and an effector organ, e.g. muscle or gland. Efferent nerve-fibres leave the spinal cord by the ventral roots.

In this book only the simple reflexes of the spinal cord (spinal reflexes) will be considered.

The receptor organ.

The receptor organ of pain, touch, or temperature sense, usually located in the skin, or a receptor organ such as the eye or ear, or a tension organ in muscle is so constructed as to be selectively responsive to agents in its environment. Thus touch and pressure receptor organs are especially responsive to mechanical stimuli, heat and cold receptor organs to changes of temperature, while other receptor organs are excited by tension in muscles [9] (Fig. 2) or by certain positions of the joints. When the stimulus to a receptor organ is strong enough, impulses are set up in the nerve-fibre connecting it to the central nervous system [2, 3, 4, 5].

It is the sole and invariable functional property of nerve-fibres to conduct 'impulses', each of which is indicated by its electrical disturbance. The only kind of nervous discharge from a receptor organ is a single impulse or train of impulses. The only modification of this discharge is by alteration of its frequency. If the frequency be high this alteration may secondarily

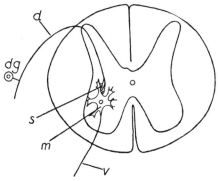

FIG. 1. A diagram of a simple reflex arc in the spinal cord. *d*, dorsal nerve-root. *v*, ventral nerve-root. *dg*, ganglion of dorsal root. *m*, motor-nerve-cell in ventral horn. *s*, region of synapse.

affect the 'size' of the impulses [131]. It is found that, within limits, when a previously inactive receptor organ is stimulated, the stronger the stimulation, the higher the frequency of its discharge. But if the stimulus be continued, the frequency gradually declines [4]. This slowing indicates that there is a progressive adjustment of the receptor organ (Fig. 3). This adjustment is termed 'adaptation' and is probably different from 'fatigue'. The rate of adaptation varies greatly in receptor organs of different type, being slowest in the tension receptors of muscle. The frequency of discharge from the organ is seldom sufficiently high for one impulse to travel in the relatively refractory period of its precursor [5, 10, 11, 131].

The afferent nerve-fibre.

The centripetal impulses set up by receptor organs traverse nerve-fibres and enter the spinal cord by the dorsal roots. Each

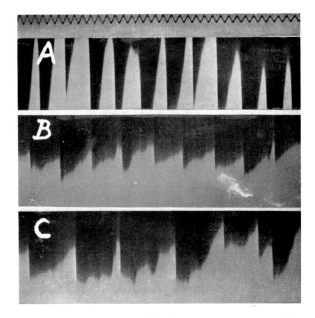

FIG. 2. Single end organ in frog's sterno-cutaneous muscle responding to stretch from a load which began to be applied 10 secs. before the photograph was taken. Time 0·01 sec. Recording instrument, capillary electrometer with 3-valve amplifier

A. load 1 grm. Responses (denoted by black shadows) are very large. Frequency of discharge 33 a second.

B. load ½ grm. Electrode distance has been reduced to diminish amplitude of excursions. Frequency 27 a second.

C. load ¼ grm. Frequency 21 a second.

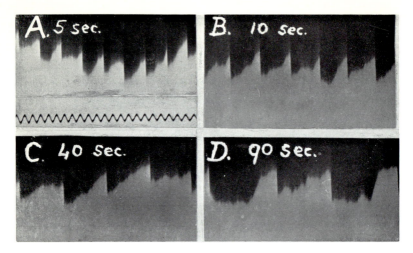

FIG. 3. Same experiment as Fig. 2. Decrease in frequency of discharge as duration of stimulus is increased. 1 grm. load.

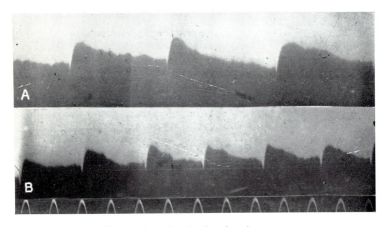

FIG. 4. Impulses in the phrenic nerve.

A. Normal breathing. Frequency of impulse, 28 a second.

B. Trachea obstructed. Frequency 50 a second.

nerve-fibre in a trunk conducts impulses independently of the other fibres. Although the precise nature of the nerve-impulse is unknown, each impulse is accompanied by an electrical disturbance which can be registered by suitable apparatus [130] (Fig. 4). The general view is that the nerve-impulse is itself an electrical phenomenon and the electrical disturbance can be regarded as a reliable measure of the impulse [60]. Under natural conditions, nerve-impulses originate from peripheral receptor organs or from nerve-cells in the central nervous system and, once started, they travel along the nerve-fibre with uniform size and speed (usually 20 to 90 metres a second). Electrical *Note* 1 stimulation of the nerve-trunk itself by the break-shock of an induction coil or by a condenser discharge is a useful artificial method of setting up nerve-impulses and it operates without loss of time. When the artificial stimulus is very weak, no nerve-impulses are set up in any of the nerve-fibres (subliminal stimulus). As the stimulus is strengthened, single nerve-impulses are set up in a few nerve-fibres (threshold or liminal stimulus). With further increases in the strength of the stimulus, single nerve-impulses are set up in more and more nerve-fibres until eventually all the fibres in the whole nerve-trunk are excited (maximal stimulus).

The aggregation of impulses set up by a single stimulus is called a single volley of impulses, or more shortly a 'single volley'. So long as the strength of the stimulus suffices to excite a nerve-fibre, the size and velocity of the impulse in that nerve-fibre are entirely independent of the strength of the stimulus. So likewise when the stimulus is repeated frequently, this independence still obtains, provided always that a sufficient period is allowed for recovery from the effects of the passage of the previous impulse. The nerve-fibre always gives its maximal response or nothing at all. This constitutes the 'all-or-nothing principle', a fundamental rule in the activity of all nerve-fibres. Nerve-impulses set up by artificial stimulation are identical with those originating from sense organs or nerve-cells. In the central as *Note* 2 well as in the peripheral nervous system there is no known form of propagation of nervous activity other than the nerve-impulse. The nerve-impulse is the universal currency of the nervous system [125, 60, 85, 91, 126].

When a nerve-impulse has travelled along a nerve-fibre, a certain period of recovery must elapse before another full-sized impulse can pass. For a short time, the 'absolutely refractory period', no stimulus, however strong, can originate an impulse. For a further interval, the 'relatively refractory period', an impulse can be set up by a stimulus stronger than that required for a rested nerve. An impulse travelling in the relatively refractory period is smaller and slower than normal [102]. In the nerves of warm-blooded animals the absolutely and relatively *Note* 3 refractory periods last for about $1.0\,\sigma$ and $5.0\,\sigma$ respectively, i.e. altogether $6.0\,\sigma$ are needed for recovery.[1] Since the total duration of the nerve-impulse as shown by the electrical disturbance is about $0.9\,\sigma$, i.e. probably a little shorter than the absolutely refractory period, it is clear that successive nerve-impulses in the same nerve-fibre must travel well spaced from one another. They cannot fuse into a steady flow, like the conduction of water in a pipe or an electric current in a wire, but may be compared to the repetitive discharge of bullets from a machine-gun.

When the stimulus to a nerve is weakened to a value below its threshold, no impulses are set up. But it may leave behind some effect, for two such stimuli in quick succession (less than $1\,\sigma$ apart) are able to excite some nerve-fibres [124]. The effectiveness of the second stimulus is due to a persistence of local change, called 'local excitatory state', which is produced by the first stimulus. The local excitatory state differs from the nerve-impulse in four respects:

(1) It is capable of summation.
(2) It is not followed by an absolutely refractory period.
(3) Its amount is proportional to the strength of the stimulus, i.e. it does not follow the all-or-nothing principle.
(4) It is not conducted along the nerve but is localized at the stimulated point.

When any single stimulus is applied to a nerve-trunk it produces a local excitatory state in each of the constituent nerve-fibres. In those where the local excitatory state is sufficiently strong, nerve-impulses are set up, but in others where the local excita-

---

[1] $1\,\sigma = 1 \times 10^{-3}$ second.

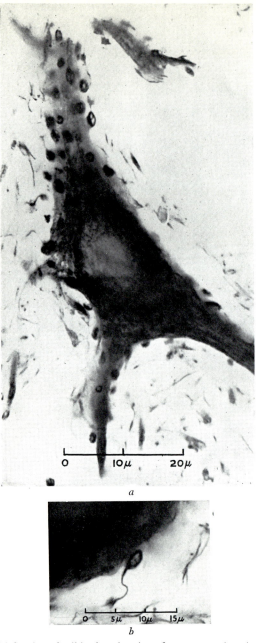

a

b

FIG. 5. (*a*) Section of cell in dorsal region of grey matter in spinal cord of
adult cat, showing 'boutons terminaux' in contact with the cell surface.
(About one hundred 'boutons' were counted on the surface of this cell,
although, of course, that number is not visible at one focus.) Compare
this figure with the model of a nerve cell shown in Fig. 202 B of ref. [95].
(*b*) Same magnification of one 'bouton' in contact with the surface of a
nerve cell of adult cat. In both these figures, the 'boutons' are somewhat
degenerated: (*a*) 43 hours, (*b*) 24 hours. [208]

tory state is too weak, no impulses are set up. In either case, the local excitatory state diminishes gradually over a period of about 1 σ. The nerve-impulse and the local excitatory state are the only excitatory conditions known to exist in peripheral nerve, and they are fundamentally similar in afferent and efferent nerve-fibres. *Note 4*

The reflex centre.

The connexion of a spinal nerve with the spinal cord by two roots, dorsal and ventral, has been described. The afferent fibres, after entering the cord, end as profuse branches on the bodies of the nerve-cells (Fig. 5 *a, b*). Although there is no accurate knowledge of the conduction of nerve-impulses along nerve-fibres and their collaterals within the spinal cord, there is no reason to suppose that it differs fundamentally from the process in peripheral nerves. Histology shows that the part of the fibre essential for conduction (axis cylinder) has a similar structure in the peripheral and central nervous systems. The actual ending of each branch is a microscopic disk, *bouton* or *pied terminal*, applied to the surface of the perikaryon, without protoplasmic connexion [44] (Fig. 5 *b*). Although accurate numbers are not available, a nerve-fibre might well be supposed to divide into branches so that it has *pieds* in varying number on the different perikarya. The surface of the perikaryon under a *pied* is a 'synapse', and this surface is almost certainly the source of the characteristic features of reflex actions. *Note 5*

The axones of the nerve-cells in the anterior horn of grey matter are the motor-nerve-fibres to muscle—hence the name of 'motoneurone' for these cells. The anterior horn cells are convergence points for reflex pathways, since the collaterals of many neurones end on their surface [190].

The effector organ.

When the efferent (motor) nerve to a muscle is stimulated, the muscle gives 'motor responses'. The afferent nerve when stimulated in the same way as the efferent nerve elicits from the muscle responses which are different from the 'motor responses' because of modification imposed by the reflex centres.

Since contraction of skeletal muscle is the only expression of functioning of reflex centres which we shall consider, the simple features of the motor response must be known before the reflex response can be compared and analysed.

A typical muscle consists of tens of thousands of muscle-fibres arranged more or less side by side and attached by one

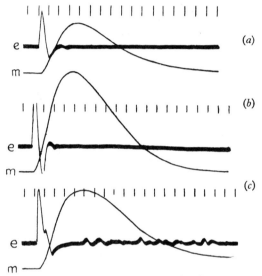

FIG. 6. Electrical *e* and mechanical *m* records of responses of tibialis anticus muscle:

(*a*). Reflex response elicited by single break-shock to popliteal nerve.

(*b*). Maximal motor twitch elicited by a single break-shock to peroneal nerve.

(*c*). As in (*a*), except that the break-shock is stronger.

Tension is shown on the scale at the side (isometrc responses). Time, 10 σ.

end to the tendon through which they pull. At the other end they are attached to bone either directly or indirectly by ten-dinous bands. On account of profuse splitting of individual nerve-fibres both just before and after entering the muscle, each motoneurone innervates on the average rather more than 100 muscle-fibres [48]. The axone of a nerve-cell together with all the muscle-fibres which it innervates by its numerous divisions is a single functional unit called the 'motor unit'. All reflexes find expression in terms of motor units.

Muscle-fibres respond by a brief contraction called a twitch when a single volley of impulses passes down the motor-nerve-fibre [57]. Such a contraction may be produced by direct electrical stimulation of the motor-nerve (motor twitch) or by impulses from the nerve-centre of the spinal cord (reflex twitch). Since the axone does not begin to divide to any great degree until it is nearing the muscle, direct stimulation of the motor-nerve-trunk excites a number of axones, and *pari passu*, according to the

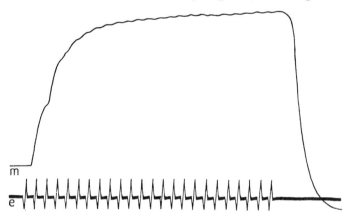

FIG. 7. Mechanical (isometric) *m* and electrical record *e* of extensor digitorum longus, motor-nerve tetanus. Rate of stimulation, 67 break-shocks a second.

strength of the current employed, the muscle-fibres innervated by them. If the stimulus is maximal, all muscle-fibres respond. Any features which are present in the reflex twitch and are absent from the motor twitch must have been added by the reflex centre (Fig. 6). When the muscle is one in which the fibres pull side by side, e.g. soleus, and not obliquely, e.g. gastrocnemius, the tension of the twitch is equal to the sum of the tensions of all the individual motor units, if care be taken to allow very little shortening. This condition is fulfilled by the isometric tension myograph, which registers optically the tension of the muscular contraction with a minimum of distortion from inertia and friction. In Fig. 6 (b) there is a typical record of a muscle twitch together with the accompanying electrical response recorded by a string galvanometer. When fewer units are excited the response is proportionately smaller and is called a submaximal twitch.

A series of volleys of impulses in the motor-nerve—no matter whether produced directly or reflexly—gives rise to an enduring muscular response, a tetanus, which continues until a short time (e.g. 30 σ) after the last volley reaches the muscle. When *Note* 6 the frequency of the volleys is not more than 70 per sec., fusion between the mechanical responses to successive volleys is not complete, and the rhythm of the responses appears in the contraction as a series of corresponding waves. The rapidly moving string of the galvanometer, on the other hand, shows that the electrical responses from the muscle are discrete (Fig. 7). The maximum tension of the tetanic contraction rises with the rate of stimulus, and when the frequency is about 60 per sec., the tetanus has a tension about four times the tension of a single twitch [57]. The tension of a tetanus or twitch for a single average motor unit is determined by dividing the tension for the whole muscle, i.e. all the motor units by the number of motor-nerve-fibres (Fig. 67) [1] which is equivalent to the number of motor units. The following values have been obtained [78]:

Tetanus.

Gastrocnemius . . .	30 grm.
Soleus	10 grm.
Extensor digitorum longus .	8 grm.
Semitendinosus . . .	6 grm.

The twitch tensions are about one-quarter of these values.

[1] See plate facing p. 99.

II

THE SPINAL GREY MATTER

THIS book is mainly concerned with spinal reflexes and their functional mechanism. It would be out of place to describe here such features of spinal structure as the long tracts in the white matter of the cord by which impulses pass to and from the higher co-ordinating centres of the brain. Yet for the understanding of reflex activities some knowledge of the minute structure of spinal white and grey matter is essential. Histological analysis [152] furnishes clues to the differences between conduction in nerve-trunks and conduction along reflex arcs. The latter are distinguished from the former by the fact that they include grey matter, with its complicated system of cell-bodies and cell-junctions, in addition to nerve-fibres.

All impulses reaching the spinal cord from the periphery enter by the dorsal (posterior) nerve-roots. Impulses passing outwards to cause contraction in skeletal muscle leave the mammalian spinal cord by the ventral (anterior) roots (Fig. 1, p. 2). The discovery of this fundamental law of the roots is due to Charles Bell (1811) and F. Magendie (1822).

The recently raised question of 'pain' afferents in the ventral roots has received a negative answer in experiments testing it in the mammalian limb [61].

According to Ingbert [110] the dorsal spinal roots on each side of a man's body contain about 634,000 myelinate fibres, and the ventral roots about 203,700. But there are, over and above these, a quantity of amyelinate small fibres in the dorsal roots the number of which has not been estimated.

The efferent fibres in the ventral roots are processes of cells whose nuclei lie in the ventral horns of grey matter. But the cell-bodies, or perikarya, of the afferent fibres are outside the *Note* 7 central nervous system in the dorsal root ganglia. It may be doubted, however, whether incoming impulses actually traverse these perikarya, since the fibres running into the cord and the fibres passing out to the periphery are united as single processes close to but outside the cell-bodies, where they thus form T-junctions. The most recent evidence [86] indicates that there is a slight delay in the passage of impulses through the ganglia. Earlier work had given conflicting results.

There is no convincing evidence that in mammals the dorsal spinal roots contain any fibres having their cells of origin elsewhere than in the root ganglia; that is, the dorsal roots contain no fibres arising within the central nervous system [133, 158, 200].

Nevin has confirmed the existence in them of amyelinate nerve-fibres. Like the more numerous myelinate fibres, they are processes of cells in the dorsal root ganglia. After section of a dorsal root between its ganglion and the spinal cord, he finds that all the fibres in the central stump degenerate. Many of the fine regenerating fibres which are later found in this situation [158] have been traced by Tower directly from the ventral roots. Tower also finds no evidence of atrophy or dystrophy in muscles that have been deafferented for several months by removal of the appropriate dorsal root ganglia [200].

Almost immediately after entering the spinal cord by a dorsal root, the afferent nerve-fibre generally, and perhaps always, splits into two, or even three, main stems (Fridtjof Nansen). One of them, the shorter, runs tailward, and the others headward, giving collaterals into the grey matter where the impulses which they convey cause either excitation or inhibition of the next neurones in the reflex arc. The course pursued by these fibres is of very variable length. Some run in the posterior columns of white matter even as far as the gracile and cuneate nuclei at the extreme top of the cord. According to current Note 8 anatomy none of the afferent root fibres or their collaterals trespass across the median longitudinal plane of the cord. A crossed reflex effect therefore involves always an internuncial neurone.

All anatomical evidence goes to show that there are no lengthy conduction paths inside the grey matter. All neurone junctions (synapses) in the cord lie in grey matter, so that a conduction path need dip into grey matter only when it is about to end. Also, every conduction path begins somewhere within the grey matter, except the path of the primary afferent neurone which starts outside the central nervous system altogether. The course of a fibre within the spinal grey matter probably never exceeds a spinal segment. An incoming fibre commonly ramifies extensively when it enters the grey matter and ends as a fine arborization in relation to a number of nerve-cells. Reflexes differ considerably in the number of successive neurones composing their arcs.

The nerve-cell (neurone) consists of a cell-body or perikaryon from which a number of cytoplasmic processes extend outwards. These processes are of two kinds. *Dendrites* are processes which branch freely close to the cell-body, and effect contact with terminal branches from other nerve-cells. They are commonly multiple, but occasionally are absent altogether. The *axone* is generally a single process, which may give off a few collaterals but typically does not ramify except near its termination. Along it impulses travel away from the cell-body either to other nerve-cells or to excitable tissues. The axis-cylinder of a motor-nerve-fibre supplying skeletal muscle, for example, is the axone of a nerve-cell the perikaryon of which is in the ventral horn of grey matter.

A recurrent collateral or 'side-fibre' given off even before such *Note 9* an axone issues from the grey matter has been observed occasionally. It has been the subject of several conjectures as to function. The absence of reflex effect from stimulation of the ventral root has to be remembered in this connexion.

When, on the other hand, the processes of a nerve-cell do *Note 10* not extend beyond the central nervous system, the axone is frequently short and almost immediately forms an arborescence (Golgi's type II). This is so in the internuncial neurones or shunt cells in the spinal grey matter.

In fixed preparations, both dendrites and axones are often found to contain numerous fine strands or *neurofibrils* running throughout their length and also continuous through the cell-body. There is some doubt whether they are present during life or are precipitation products caused by fixation. Many investigators have looked for them in vain in living vertebrate nerve-cells. In any case it seems difficult to regard them as the 'units' of nervous conduction, since a nerve-fibre *as a whole* obeys the all-or-nothing law [15].

In the *perikaryon* is found the nucleus, containing a well-marked nucleolus. This part of the cell possesses other interesting cytological features. Mitochondria are present in its cytoplasm, together with peculiar angular structures, staining well with methylene blue, known as *Nissl granules*.   The latter may perhaps be artefacts due to the fixatives employed, but nevertheless they must have some precursor in the living cell; so that, even if they should prove to be post-mortem phenomena, their distribution and properties would still be worthy of attention. They are absent from the axone-hillock (or that part of the cell-body in which the efferent fibre originates) but may be found in the proximal portions of the dendrites.   Under various conditions, such as after prolonged stimulation, they tend to disappear.   They also suffer disintegration or 'chromatolysis' *Note* 11 when their cell is mutilated by section of one of its processes. When examined during life by micro-dissection methods, the protoplasm of the perikaryon is found to be highly viscid (Chambers).

Another structure present in the cell-body, and which shows characteristic changes when a nerve-fibre is cut, is the *Golgi apparatus*, a reticulum which finds its most complex development in the cytoplasm of nerve-cells.   The changes which it undergoes are displacement to the periphery of the cell or 'retispersion', often followed by fragmentation or 'retisolution'. This structure has been shown [136] to be entirely separate from a canalicular system found in nerve-cells and named after its discoverer Holmgren.   The two can be demonstrated as separate morphological entities in the same nerve-cell, and the latter exhibits no alteration during retispersion.   Their functions are unknown.

The discovery that the direction of conduction through a nerve-cell could be confidently inferred from the microscopic appearance of the cell was made by Cajal and van Gehuchten independently, when they showed that the sense of conduction was always cellulipetal in dendrites, cellulifugal in axones.

Nerve-cells are to be regarded as the anatomical units of which the nervous system is built. Although the most characteristic feature of the nervous system is its ability to transmit propagated disturbances from one part of the body to another, and this conduction almost invariably involves a whole series of neurones, the individual nerve-cell is, nevertheless, in several respects quite independent of its fellows.   The plexus of nerve-processes in grey matter does not constitute a syncytium. The facts of degeneration prove each neurone to be a self-contained independent anatomical unit. In accordance with the general rule, any part of a nerve-cell which is severed from its nucleus degenerates. Thus, after division of a peripheral nerve-trunk, the axis-cylinders of all fibres distal to the section die and are absorbed. On the central side of the point of section the fibres usually remain healthy. When the spinal cord is cut, the pyramidal and other descending tracts exhibit a similar atrophy below the level of the transection. But Wallerian degeneration does not extend to processes of other cells, for instance, the ventral horn cells, with which these tracts communicate only functionally. Chromatolysis and retispersion have been mentioned as occurring in the perikarya of mutilated cells. Below a transection of the cord, these changes are conspicuous in the cells of Clarke's column, from which important ascending tracts arise, but they are not seen in the motor-cells of the ventral horn.

The Golgi silver method also shows discontinuity between nerve-cells. Only a small proportion of the cells in a preparation take up the stain, but a singularly clear picture is obtained of all the ramifying processes of such as do. These processes are never seen to fuse with the processes or cell-bodies of other nerve-cells. They end merely in close apposition to the latter.

Finally, the irreversibility of conduction through grey matter seems inexplicable except in terms of a definite surface of separation, or polarized membrane, between nerve-cell and nerve-cell. Nerve-fibres are known to conduct impulses equally well in either direction, whereas no reflex movement can be evoked by stimulation of the central stump of a cut ventral spinal root. This 'law of forward direction' cannot well be attributed to the cell-bodies contained in grey matter, since dorsal root ganglia conduct in both directions. Nor, as we have seen, is it a property of those cell-processes which are met with in peripheral nerve. The junctions between successive neurones are the only other structures interpolated in the reflex arc to which we can ascribe such blockage of 'antidromic' conduction.

The minute structure of these points of contact between

nerve-cells, 'synapses', is by no means easy to determine, because shrinkage and distortion of the very delicate elements involved must inevitably accompany fixation, imbedding, and staining, Fig. 5 *a, b*. The 'boutons terminaux' (Cajal) which form the terminal arborizations of axones in grey matter, are applied to the surface both of the dendrites and of the perikarya of other neurones [44]. If we confine our attention to the junction between only two successive neurones, there are not one but many points of contact across which influences can be exerted. A further conspicuous feature is that one neurone is usually connected functionally with a considerable number of others next 'down-stream' to it, while these latter are themselves each subject to the influence of several next 'up-stream' neurones. Here we find the anatomical basis (*a*) for the experimental finding that a reflex response is rarely, if ever, confined to a single effector unit, and (*b*) for the principle of convergence of many afferent arcs on a single 'final common path'.

Histological analysis thus reveals a feature of the reflex arc differing qualitatively from anything found in a nerve-trunk. Correspondingly we shall see in subsequent chapters that impulses do not pass direct from nerve-cell to nerve-cell, but that at each relay a fresh set of impulses is set up, provided the excitatory process attains there a threshold value.

So also in the sympathetic ganglia there is no direct anatomical continuity of pre-ganglionic neurone with post-ganglionic. Conduction through these ganglia [144] resembles that through reflex arcs in that there is often no close correspondence between rhythm of stimulus and rhythm of response.

The anatomical evidence that there is contact but not continuity between the successive links in a connected chain of neurones is entirely consistent with the facts which we shall have before us in this book. So far as is known, however, no clear morphological difference distinguishes the 'boutons' into two classes, although, as we shall see later, central excitation and central inhibition are two distinct processes occurring in the spinal grey matter.

The question whether the connexion between successive neurones is one of mere contact or of actual structural continuity is of much interest for function. Histologists have sometimes doubted Cajal's

view that the 'boutons terminaux' represent truly the mode of connexion between one neurone and another. They have claimed that
the 'boutons' may be coagulated intercellular matrix drawn into
fibrils during the shrinking of the cell, or that they may be terminations of neuroglia fibres. The evidence to the contrary seems conclusive. Tiegs [198, 199] describes that between two nerve-cells there
is protoplasmic continuity, and not mere contiguity. In fixed preparations of the cord, he describes axone-collaterals branching freely
in grey matter and finally penetrating dendrites. The neurofibrils,
he says, pass without interruption from cell to cell. He and others
have described neurofibrils as being occasionally visible 'in unfixed
and apparently living nerve-cells'; and 'histological research leads'
him 'to the conclusion that the neurofibril, rather than the neurone,
is the elementary conducting unit of the nervous system'. The
majority of histological observers favour the discontinuity view.
Even the nervous system of Medusa, usually cited as an instance of
continuity, was shown by Schäfer, as long ago as 1878 [151], to consist of an interlacement of nerve-cells and their filaments which are
discrete and nowhere continuous one with another nor united into a
network. This observation has recently been confirmed [21].

In some of its properties, grey matter exhibits differences of
degree rather than of kind in comparison with nerve-trunks.
Examples are the great susceptibility of the former to fatigue
and asphyxia, and to the action of such drugs as chloroform,
nicotine, and strychnine. The site of incidence of these influences is still undetermined. They may act at the synapses by
altering the condition of the surface of separation or by changing
the excitability of the down-stream neurones. On the other
hand, emphasis has been laid, especially by Lucas [125], Adrian,
Forbes [89], and Hill [106], on the extremely fine non-medullated nerve-filaments by which impulses are conducted in grey
matter. They are threads much more slender than even the
most slender medullated fibres in the peripheral nerve-trunks or
white columns of the cord. Judging from analogy the speed of
conduction for impulses in these fibres must be slower than the
slowest conduction in nerve-trunks or in white matter. Their
length, however, is always short. It may well be that the ex-   *Note 12*
planation for many of the features characteristic of reflex arcs
is to be found in the properties of these structures. In particular, they are of interest in regard to the 'central time' of reflexes

(p. 19). In keeping with the proneness of grey matter to fatigue and asphyxia is the richness of its blood-supply as compared with that of white matter.

The final link in the path through which reflex contraction is evoked in skeletal muscle is formed by the large motoneurones in the ventral horns of grey matter. The axones of these cells conduct impulses direct to the muscles. Such an axone, together with the muscle-fibres which it innervates, therefore constitutes the effector unit in reflex response. The whole is accordingly termed a 'motor unit'. It may contain as many as 160 muscle-fibres [48]. In order to innervate so many muscle-fibres, nerve-fibres branch very extensively in the substance of the muscle which they supply. Sometimes also dichotomous division is met with in motor-nerve-fibres at a distance from the muscle [49, 78]. Muscle-fibres show rapid atrophy when the axone supplying them is cut or when their motoneurone dies. An exception to this rule is provided by the intrafusal muscle-fibres in muscle-spindles. They alone fail to degenerate when a motor-nerve is severed.

III

THE FLEXOR REFLEX

Introduction.

A SIMPLE field for investigating reflex action is the lower part of the spinal cord after its isolation from the rest of the central nervous system by transection at the lower thoracic or upper lumbar level. This isolated portion of the spinal cord is capable of certain elementary reflexes of which the following is an example. A dog, whose spinal cord has been transected several days before, is lifted off the ground. Its hind limbs remain flaccid and show no spontaneous activity. If, however, one paw is pricked by a needle, there will be a sudden withdrawal of the limb because the flexor muscles of the hip, knee, and ankle contract. The contraction may continue for several seconds and then gradually subsides. Just as in the frog (p. 1), so in the dog, destruction of the isolated portion of the cord or section of the dorsal or ventral roots abolishes all responses. The function of this type of reflex, the flexor reflex, is to withdraw the limb from contact with injurious agents. The long continuation of the response is not conditioned by the contracting muscle itself, for when contraction is brought about by stimulation of the motor-nerve, the muscle relaxes very quickly afterwards. To what cause can the delay in relaxation be ascribed—to a cause on the afferent side of the reflex arc or to a cause in the reflex centre? Pain from a prick, be it remembered, lasts for some time, and Adrian has shown that with a prick there is a prolonged discharge of impulses in the afferent nerve [3], therefore the sustained character of the withdrawal may be dependent on the continued arrival of such impulses. How much of the prolonged discharge is due to this cause and how much to some activity in reflex centres has not yet been decided by any direct method. Electrical stimulation of afferent nerves, however, throws light on the relative contribution from any central source.[1]

[1] Although stimulation of nerve-trunks is convenient in practice, one must *Note* 13 not lose sight of the fact that it does not occur under natural conditions. In the nerve-trunk, fibres of the most diverse function, e.g. pain, touch, temperature sense, &c., are all excited together so that the reflex centres are subjected to a volley of impulses of widely different reflex significance and their co-ordinating function is thereby severely taxed.

Note 14   No more than one single propagated disturbance is set up in any nerve-fibre by the application of a single stimulus to the nerve-trunk, e.g. by the break-shock of an induction coil [1] or by the discharge of a condenser of small capacity, unless the stimulus is very strong. If then a single weak stimulus be applied to a suitable afferent nerve, the resulting single volley of centripetal impulses produces a reflex response of very short duration. In fact the response may appear as rapid as the twitch produced by stimulation of the motor-nerve. To make accurate observation of this twitch, the tendon of a chosen flexor muscle is attached to the myograph, while all other muscles are immobilized by denervation, and the bones of the limb are fixed rigidly by drills. In its general features, as has been said, the myographic record of the reflex response is very similar to the motor twitch (Fig. 6, *a* and *b*). The simultaneous record of the string galvanometer shows that the action-current of the muscle during the reflex response is also very similar to that of a motor twitch except that the responses of individual motor units are more spread out in time, the volley of reflex impulses having a temporal dispersion sometimes 3 σ or longer. Even with a temporal dispersion of this order there is often only a single impulse discharged from each motoneurone. When this is the case, the resulting muscular contraction is said to be a *reflex twitch* [79]. It can be distinguished from a submaximal motor twitch of similar tension only by its greater temporal dispersion.

When the stimulus to the afferent nerve is weaker, centripetal impulses are set up in fewer afferent fibres, and so the resulting reflex response is smaller. If the centripetal impulses are very few in number, there may even be no reflex response. On the other hand, when the stimulus to the afferent nerve is made stronger, more afferent fibres are excited and the resulting reflex *Note* 15 response is larger. Above a certain strength of stimulus a stage is reached when the reflex response changes its character, and both the mechanical and electrical records show that the reflex discharge continues for some time after the first large initial volley. Since the strength of stimulus requisite for eliciting such an enduring discharge is too weak to give rise to more than

---

[1] Without an iron core, for this delays the rate of demagnetization of the system and so prolongs the break-induced current.

one impulse in any afferent nerve-fibre, the prolonged discharge of the reflex response must originate in the reflex centres. This prolongation is, in fact, a common characteristic of this and other reflexes and it occurs, as we have seen, when a single volley of impulses in a sufficiently large number of afferent fibres impinges on the centre. In the flexor reflex, the discharge may last 100σ or longer (Fig. 6, c). This 'after-discharge', as it is called, is not due to the muscle re-exciting itself reflexly by impulses initiated in its own receptor organs as a result of the contraction [13], for the discharge obtains also in the deafferented preparation. After-discharge, therefore, must be the discharge of impulses from the reflex centres which continues after withdrawal of the external stimulus. During this or any other central activity several impulses may be discharged from a single motoneurone, and the impulses from any one motoneurone are likely to be 'out of step', i.e. out of phase with the impulses from other motoneurones.

Latent Period.

If the moment of stimulation be registered, it will be seen that there is a considerable delay—'latent period'—before the efferent discharge signals its arrival in the muscle by the start of the action current. Part of this delay can be calculated and allowed for as the time needed for the passage of centripetal impulses to the cord [1] and from there to the muscle. When these times are subtracted from the total latent period the remaining interval—the 'central reflex time'—represents the passage through the cord [79, 90, 111]. In the example below this period is estimated by taking the time of arrival of the centrifugal volley at a point in the motor-nerve so that the latent period of the muscular response need not be considered.

	σ
Time for passage of impulses in 13·8 cm. of afferent nerve at 31·6 metres a second*	4·4
Time for passage of impulses in 19·5 cm. of efferent nerve at 93 metres a second*	2·1
∴ Total time for peripheral path	6·5
Apparent latent period observed	10·4
∴ Central reflex time	3·9

* The actual rates are determined at the same time as the main experiment.

[1] No appreciable time is occupied by the break-shock in setting up the centripetal volley.

In general, the flexor reflex has a central reflex time between
3·0 and 5·5 σ.

The weaker the stimulus which is applied to an afferent
nerve, the longer is the latent period of the resulting reflex
response. This is shown in Fig. 8, where the tension of the
reflex response (ordinates) is plotted against the latent period
(abscissae). Spread of the stimulating current along the afferent
nerve can only account for a very small part of this alteration of

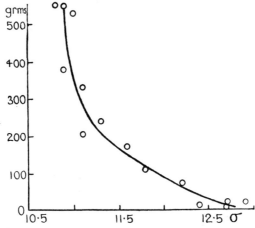

FIG. 8. The tensions of a series of reflex responses (ordinates) are plotted
against their respective latent periods (abscissae). Tibialis anticus muscle
reflexly excited from ipselateral popliteal nerve.

the latent period. For example in Fig. 8, although the strength
of the stimulus was progressively weakened more during the
series of six observations with the shortest latent period than it
was for all the remaining observations of the series, the latent
period lengthened only 0·3 σ for these six observations as against
1·8 σ for the remainder of the series.

The lengthening of latent period therefore is almost entirely
due to an increase in the central reflex time of the reflex
responses evoked by smaller centripetal volleys.

Reflex Tetanus.

When an ipselateral afferent nerve is subjected to repetitive
stimulation there ensues in the flexor muscle a prolonged con-

traction, which in many respects resembles a motor tetanus. The rise of reflex tension is as steep as in the motor response of the same frequency. This rapid rise in the reflex shows that all the motor units engaged respond to the first stimulus of the series. Reflexes of this type are called 'd'emblée' reflexes [117]. As long as the stimulus is continued, the tension of the 'motor' tetanus is fairly well maintained although often it shows a slight progressive decline. On the other hand, the reflex tetanus is

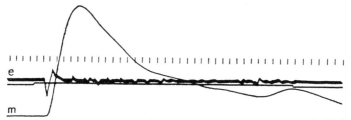

FIG. 9. Electrical *e* and mechanical *m* records of responses of tibialis anticus muscle elicited by repetitive stimulation of popliteal nerve. The response rapidly falls off during the continuation of the stimulation. Time, 10 σ.

more variable. It may, on occasion, rise slowly for a time, but often it declines quite early and abruptly, Fig. 9.

The rhythm of the reflex response [116].

Note 16

When the frequency of the centripetal volleys is lower than 50 per sec., the rhythm is just visible in the myogram of the tetanus as small undulations, Fig. 10. In the motor tetanus, however, this rate of stimulation gives a clearly defined rhythm. Why then is the rhythm blurred in the reflex response? The answer is found by studying the electrical record of the response, which shows small accessory action-currents between the main volleys of the rhythm [50]. These small electrical responses, 'secondary waves' (Fig. 10, *c*), are due to after-discharge from the preceding stimulus. They maintain the mechanical tension of the muscle between the main volleys and tend to produce a smooth tetanus.

Further comparison between motor and reflex responses [117].

Blurring of the rhythm in the plateau of the reflex is not the only evidence of modification imposed by the motoneurones.

If Fig. 10 *a*, *b*, is carefully examined, it will be noticed that the first step is higher in the reflex than in the motor tetanus. That is to say, the first volley of impulses from the reflex centre pro-

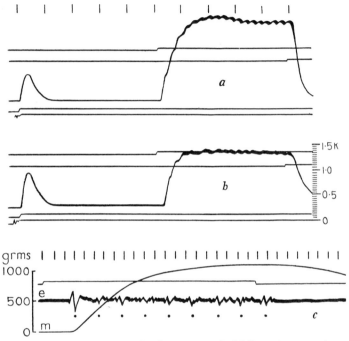

FIG. 10. Myographic records of responses of tibialis anticus muscle set up as follows:

(*a*) Motor responses elicited by a single break-shock followed by a tetanic stimulation at frequency of 39 per sec.

(*b*) Reflex responses elicited by a single break-shock to the ipselateral popliteal nerve followed by a tetanic stimulation at a frequency of 39 per sec. Time, 0·1 sec.

(*c*) Electrical *e* and mechanical *m* records of the response of tibialis anticus muscle to a repetitive stimulation of posterior tibial nerve. The secondary waves can be seen as small undulations between the primary waves which are marked by dots underneath. Time, 10 σ.

duces greater effective activity in the muscle-fibres than the first volley from direct stimulation of the motor-nerve. Asynchronism of the centrifugal volley by itself would not produce the higher step, but repetitive firing of the centre would. Therefore, even at its first outburst, the centre shows repetitive firing

('after-discharge'). When the first step of the reflex is compared with the ultimate height, the ratio is usually 1 : 2·5 (ratio
of single shock : tetanus), though in Fig. 10, *a*, *b*, the ratio is
nearer 1 : 2. In some cases the low ratio is due to ipselateral
inhibition. On the other hand, the first step of the motor
response may be 1 : 3 or 1 : 4 of the total height.

When the series of tetanic stimuli comes to an end, the motor
response subsides fairly rapidly, but the reflex response subsides slowly and reaches the base line much later, because the
repetitive after-discharge of the centre continues for some time
after the withdrawal of the stimulus. In the deafferented
preparation, however, the after-discharge is very much reduced.

Fractionation of the reflex centre [51].

If a series of records be made with progressive increase in the
number of afferent fibres tetanically stimulated at a rate of
50 per sec., it is found that increase of the strength of
stimulus beyond a certain intensity fails to augment the tension of the reflex. The reflex is then a maximal reflex for that
particular afferent nerve. It might, of course, be suspected that
the maximum is reached only because all the motor units of the
muscle are reflexly excited, and the maximal reflex, *ceteris
paribus*, might equal the maximal motor response. But, in fact,
the tension of the maximal motor response usually far exceeds
that of the maximal reflex response. Hence one must conclude
that only a fraction of the motor units usually take part in the
reflex response elicited from any one afferent nerve, and it is
probable that the maximum reflex is reached for any particular
afferent nerve only when each stimulus is strong enough to
excite all the constituent afferent fibres.

This fractional participation of units according to the nerve
selected can be seen in Table I.

Here, in the same preparation, the number of motor units
involved varies according to the afferent nerve selected, but any
particular nerve excites almost the same proportion of units of
the same flexor in one animal as in another. Assessing the tetanic
contraction-value of the average motor unit of tibialis anticus
at 8 grm. [78], the number of units at the disposal of each of
the above several afferent nerves can be tentatively given, e.g.

for external plantar not less than 155 motor units. Among
different flexors, however, the proportion does vary, e.g. the
popliteal nerve excites only 28 per cent. of tensor fasciae femoris,
but about 80 per cent. of semitendinosus and tibialis anticus.
As a rule, small or segmentally remote afferent nerves command
only a small fraction, e.g. internal saphenous and obturator
nerves for tibialis anticus, Table I. On the other hand, there
are small nerves which excite a notably large fraction, e.g. the
dorsal digital nerves individually may excite as much as 80 per
cent. of semitendinosus.

TABLE I.

M. Tibialis Anticus.   Maximum motor tension 2160 grammes.

Afferent nerve stimulated.	Tension of maximal reflex tetanus in grammes.	Reflex tension expressed as percentage of maximal motor tetanus.
Internal saphenous . . .	800	32
Superficial obturator . .	165	6·7
Deep obturator . . .	400	16
Nerve to quadriceps and sartorius	1190	44
Musculo-cutaneous branch of peroneal	1700	69
External plantar . . .	1240	50
Internal plantar . . .	1330	54
Small sciatic	680	28
Hamstring	565	23
Nerve of sural triceps . .	300 (rather low)	12
Total	8370	

Note 17   The fraction of motoneurones reflexly excited by an afferent
nerve alters during the course of an experiment. As a rule there
is a gradual increase due, probably, to recovery from spinal
shock after transection of the cord, although at first recovery
from anaesthesia cannot be neglected. In weak preparations
fatigue or a failing blood-supply may cause continued fluctuations. Strychnine too, in subconvulsive doses, alters the size of
the fraction which is accessible, but the fraction does not reach
unity. These results point to there being a limit to the size of
fraction accessible to an afferent nerve. If strict anatomical
limitations existed, there would be no transient fluctuations.

Principle of Convergence.

From Table I it is clear that the sum of the tensions of the reflex responses of a muscle elicited from individual afferent nerves far exceeds the maximal motor tension which can be developed by stimulation of the motor-nerve. This can only mean that some motor units are excited from more than one afferent nerve. The central terminations of different afferent nerves must therefore converge on to the same motoneurone. Hence arises an overlap of their respective reflex fields. This 'Principle of Convergence' [164, 168] is the basis of co-ordinated function in the nervous system. Myographic evidence for multiple convergence is strongly supported by histological study of the central nervous system, which emphasizes the wealth of convergence in the reflex pathways of the spinal cord.

If, instead of using the main nerves mentioned in Table I, one stimulates separately the several tributary nerves composing them, the aggregate reflex tension exceeds that from the intact main nerve, and values of more than seven times the maximal motor tetanus have been obtained under such conditions. A central functional convergence as great as this gives a glimpse of the degree of overlap which the microscope shows to exist within the central nervous system.[1] Even small nerves contain hundreds of afferent fibres with consequent possibilities of intense convergence, and these possibilities are multiplied by the existence of many collaterals which are given off by each afferent nerve after entering the spinal cord.

Occlusion [45, 52].

Another aspect of this overlapping distribution has been brought to light by setting up concurrently a series of centripetal volleys in two afferent nerves. When, for example, tibialis anticus muscle is excited reflexly by concurrent stimulation of two plantar nerves, the reflex tension is more, e.g. 1·81 kg., than when one plantar nerve alone is stimulated, e.g. 1·57 kg., but is *much less* than the sum produced by adding the tensions from stimulation of the nerves separately, e.g. 1·57 + 1·58 kg. (Fig. 11).

[1] Peripheral convergence due to branching of peripheral afferent nerve-fibres is negligible, but see Adrian, Cattell, and Hoagland [7].

This result is what would be anticipated from our knowledge of overlap, for the motor units common to both nerves are already excited maximally by one nerve so far as the development of tension is concerned. The centripetal volleys, therefore, from the second nerve cannot cause the development of any extra tension. The consequent deficit of tension is called 'Occlusion'. In the above example the occlusion amounts to

$$1\cdot57 + 1\cdot58 - 1\cdot81 \text{ kg.} = 1\cdot34 \text{ kg.}$$

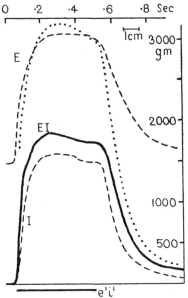

FIG. 11. Contractions of tibialis anticus muscle evoked as follows:
Upper broken line—from tetanic stimulation of external plantar nerve alone during $e'i'$. (For clearness, this upper line is drawn 1·5 kg. above its actual tension.)
Lower broken line—similarly for internal plantar nerve alone.
Dotted line—the course of the contraction if these two contractions had fully added themselves during concurrent stimulation of both nerves.
Continuous line—the actual response obtained under these conditions.

It may be argued that the lack of added contraction during overlap is due to the motoneurones being already so fully excited by one nerve that impulses arriving from the other nerve are for some reason ineffective for exciting them further. This objection cannot be met from the record of muscular tension alone, because, of course, the muscular units are already excited maximally. But the objection can be met from the electrical record [56] which shows that the rhythm of the muscular action-currents and therefore of the motoneurone discharge is double, and that the motoneurones are responding to both series of centripetal volleys (provided always that one series of responses is not prevented by the refractory periods of the other series). Both series of centripetal volleys do therefore activate the motoneurones.

Possibly part of the contraction-deficit in the concurrent response may be due to inhibition. Against that likelihood is the fact that, although in cases where the convergent afferents are large there would be a special risk of it, and, although the contraction-deficit is heavy, no trace of effective inhibition exists because there is a maximal tetanic contraction of the whole muscle.

It is convenient to have a simple diagram to represent the effects of overlap between the motor units excited by centri-

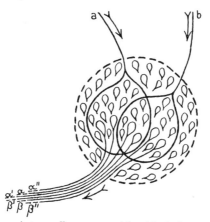

FIG. 12. Two excitatory afferents, a and b, with their respective fields of threshold excitation in the motoneurone pool of a muscle. Axones are drawn for only four of the motoneurones activated by a alone (a'', a, a', and β') and by b alone (β', β, β'', and a'). Concurrently they activate not eight but six, i.e. give a contraction deficit by occlusion of contraction in a' and β'.

petal volleys in different nerves. In Fig. 12 the anterior horn cells which correspond to the motor units of a muscle are set inside a circle. This is the 'motor centre' of the muscle or its 'motoneurone pool'. The fractional portions excited to discharge by centripetal volleys in reflexes a and b are shown as small areas circumscribed by the continuation of the line representing the nerve in question, and each can be referred to as the motoneurone field of that nerve. For simplicity in the diagram, only six neurones are supposed to be concerned. Each motoneurone may be assumed, for the purposes of argument, to have the same tension value in the myogram. Four of these motoneurones are in the field of nerve a and four in the field of b, so that two are common to both. If a tetanic reflex is elicited by nerve *a*, nerve *b* can, *ceteris paribus*, add in the myogram only the tension of two more units. This is only half its reflex effect when alone. In other words, reflex *b* has suffered a 50 per cent. occlusion by reflex *a*. Similarly, a series of volleys in *a* nerve during the reflex from *b* nerve show an occlusion of *a* reflex by *b* reflex.

Occlusion therefore is a measure of central overlap. The more motor units which two reflexes have in common, the greater will be the opportunity for occlusion. Occlusion exists not only between reflexes from closely allied nerves, e.g. the two plantar nerves, but also between reflexes from nerves most diverse segmentally and functionally, e.g. the external cutaneous nerve of groin and the hamstring nerve, or the internal saphenous nerve and the nerve to sartorius. Hence the wide range of convergence of paths within the cord must again be emphasized as showing how co-ordination of function can be attained.

As the amount of occlusion between reflexes from closely allied nerves, e.g. two plantar or two dorsal digital nerves, is usually greater than one would expect from the size of the independent reflexes, the motoneurone fields excited by such a pair of nerves must be very similar—an important factor in the co-ordination of function. Fig. 12 leads one to expect that the more extensive the motoneurone field in one reflex, the greater the occlusion of any other reflex. This does occur, for if tibialis anticus is observed, its response to weak centripetal volleys in the internal plantar nerve occludes less than 80 per cent. of the response from the external plantar nerve, but with increase in the strength of the volleys the occlusion is nearly 95 per cent. [52]. A very powerful reflex may occlude another completely.

Conversely, decrease of the motoneurone field by reducing the size of centripetal volleys, by spinal shock or by fatigue, reduces the amount of occlusion. Weak reflex responses may show no occlusion at all, and under some circumstances the conjoint effect of the two reflexes may be greater than the sum of the two acting independently. This phenomenon occurs because the two series of centripetal volleys, when concurrent, activate some motor units which are not activated by either series alone. This is an example of facilitation, the outcome of which is the reverse of occlusion.

When facilitation occurs in strong reflexes it is masked by occlusion. During the concurrence of centripetal volleys, the addition of a few motor units by facilitation makes a tension deficiency from occlusion appear less than it really is. Any error from this source is probably small enough to be neglected when maximal stimuli are employed. More important than such facilitation is the inhibitory effect which impulses in one nerve may exert upon the excitation from the other [52, 80]. As this is incomplete and associated also with some excitatory effect, it may be difficult to detect and the tension deficiency due to occlusion may be over-estimated. In powerful reflexes, complication from inhibition may be absent. For instance, when one powerful reflex is occluded by another one still more powerful, every motor unit of the muscle may be found in action.

When two series of centripetal volleys evoke concurrent reflexes, their temporal relationship merits consideration. For example, both may begin and end together, or one may be intercurrent for a short time during the other or one may start sooner and finish sooner. All types are equally suitable for demonstrating occlusion, but the last two have the advantage of showing its beginning and end. Occlusion, of course, begins when the intercurrent reflex begins. During the concurrence of the two reflexes, the contraction plateau of the myogram is maintained more steadily than when one reflex alone is operative. Each reflex steadies and sustains the other in those central paths which they activate in common. On cessation of one reflex the other reflex is usually left without any obvious trace of the concurrence. Since the electrical record shows that each reflex continues independently of the other except for the influence of the refractory period of the common path, it can be understood why one reflex as a general rule emerges so little affected from occlusion. An exception occurs if the emerging reflex is of the 'jet' type which shows a very rapid decline of tension (Fig. 9), for then it is often better sustained after a short period of concurrence with some other reflex.

The reflex field of flexors of a whole limb. Fractionation.

Thus far we have been concerned with the influence of centripetal volleys of impulses in various afferent nerves upon the reflex centre of a single flexor muscle (tibialis anticus, semi-tendinosus, or tensor fasciae femoris). But the flexor reflex is not confined to a single muscle, as our preliminary example showed, nor to the flexor muscles of a single joint, but in greater or less degree to all the flexor muscles of all joints—hip, knee, and ankle [178]. In the study of the reflex responses of one muscle we have neglected the wider distribution of the reflex. Nevertheless, those three muscles which have been observed at different times are types of hip, knee, and ankle flexors, so that the results on occlusion and fractionation may be assumed to hold for all flexor muscles.

Experiments on fractionation show that there is often variation in the fractions of various muscles reflexly excited by maximal centripetal volleys in one nerve. By taking records simultaneously of the reflex contractions of two muscles in response to centripetal volleys in one nerve, it is possible to get a further knowledge of reflex co-ordination among flexor muscles [58].

In Table II, for example, the tensions of the reflex responses for each nerve are expressed as percentages of the strongest contraction.

TABLE II.

Nerve.	Hip flexor. (Tens. fasciae fem.)	Knee flexor. (Semitendin.)	Ankle flexor. (Tib. ant.)
Int. saph. . .	100	56	87
Popliteal . .	3 or less	42	100
Peroneal distal to Tib. ant. n. .	14	100	69

The reflex field excited by centripetal volleys in any nerve is distributed in a characteristic manner over fractions of the centres of all the flexor muscles of the limb. These fractions depend largely on functional conditions such as spinal shock, fatigue, and blood-supply, but there is an underlying basis of anatomical significance.

In any nerve the centripetal volleys which are just strong enough to evoke a reflex response in one muscle, are sufficient for other muscles, that is, the thresholds are the same. Each step of increasing the number of active afferent fibres, that is, the number of centripetal impulses, increases the absolute amount of reflex contraction by activating more motor units, although the ratio of the responses of any two muscles is usually altered. Different muscles have almost identical latent periods for their reflex responses. Thus in fractional involvement, in threshold, and in latent period different flexor muscles have the same characteristics in response to a particular series of centripetal volleys. The reflex field which can be excited by centripetal volleys from any nerve includes those fractionated groups of flexor motor units which are bound together by functional similarities of threshold and latent period. The reflex field is a functional entity including extensor as well as flexor muscles, unrestricted by anatomical boundaries such as the limits of the motoneurone centre of any particular muscle, although, owing to the greater involvement of some centres, each nerve has its own characteristic field. The term flexor reflex, therefore, denotes a group of reflexes which employ similar muscles but in the detailed distribution of motor units differ one from another.

THE REFLEX RESPONSE EVOKED BY TWO
CENTRIPETAL VOLLEYS

(a) *When each is just too weak to evoke a reflex response. Summation.*

If the stimuli (single break-shocks) applied to two afferent nerves are reduced so that either alone is just too weak to elicit a reflex response, there may be a small response when the stimuli are applied at a short interval apart [25, 27, 77, 190]. The reflex response is the smaller the longer the interval, and disappears when the stimuli are separated by a sufficiently long interval. Thus in Fig. 13 each point denotes the tension developed by the reflex contraction of tibialis anticus in response to stimuli applied to the medial and lateral nerves to gastrocnemius at the interval indicated.

After exclusion of other tentative explanations, we are left with the explanation that the reflex response must be due to summation within the spinal cord [77]. Either stimulus alone sets up a centripetal volley which is unable to evoke a reflex discharge, but at short stimulus-intervals the excitatory condition produced by one volley sums with that produced by the other and sets up a reflex discharge from some motoneurones. The smaller response at any longer stimulus-interval indicates that a discharge has been evoked from fewer motoneurones. Therefore, in some motoneurones, the excitatory condition remaining from the first volley is added to that produced by the second volley and reaches a threshold intensity at a short, but not at a long, interval. Similar arguments applied to a series of observations make it possible to conclude that in any moto-

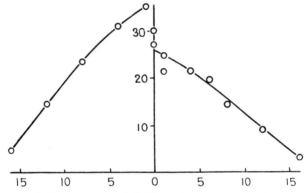

FIG. 13. Reflex responses of tibialis anticus to two stimuli (each one of which alone is just threshold) to med. gastroc. n. and lat. gastroc. n. at various intervals. Abscissae, stimulus interval in sigmata, ordinates tension in grams. To right of zero, lat. gastroc. n. is stimulated first, to left of zero, med. gastroc. n. first. Curve shows relation of resulting tension to stimulus interval.

neurone the excitatory condition (if subliminal) produced by a centripetal volley diminishes progressively in intensity until at a sufficiently long interval no trace can be detected. The enduring excitatory condition thus set up by a centripetal volley can be conveniently called the central excitatory state, c.e.s., without prejudice as to its precise nature.

There is a summation of the central effects of centripetal volleys in different afferent nerves and it follows that such afferent pathways must converge upon the same motoneurones. For example in Fig. 14, if the motoneurones enclosed by the afferent paths a and b be supposed each to represent the respective fields of subliminal excitation, then summation of c.e.s. is possible only in those motoneurones common to each field.

Summation probably occurs at the actual convergence points on the motoneurones rather than during the passage along common nerve paths, e.g. in overcoming a block from decremental conduction, for in the latter case one would expect some evidence of a refractory period following the first centripetal volley. But no such evidence exists.

When centripetal impulses reach this part of a motoneurone they suffer a change whereby they become capable of summa-

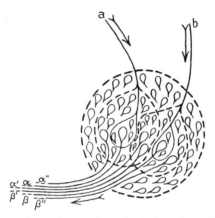

FIG. 14. As in Fig. 12 but weaker stimulation of *a* and *b* restricts the respective fields of threshold excitation as shown by the continuous line limit. *a* by itself activates 1 unit a; *b* similarly β. Concurrently they activate 4 units (a', a, β', and β) owing to summation of the subliminal effect in the overlap of the subliminal fields outlined by the dots. (Subliminal fields of effect are not indicated in Fig. 12.)

tion, i.e. they are transformed into so much *c.e.s.* which, if sufficiently intense, sets up a reflex discharge passing as a nerve-impulse down the axone of the motoneurone. If the *c.e.s.* fails to set up a reflex discharge, i.e. is subliminal, it diminishes progressively until none is detectable after a period of, usually, 10 σ to 20 σ.

As might be expected, there is also summation of the effects of two centripetal volleys which are set up in the same afferent nerve. If, however, the stimuli are applied to the nerve at too short an interval the centripetal volley set up by the second stimulus will be small or absent owing to the refractory period of the afferent nerve-fibres, which follows the first volley. For this reason the reflex response elicited by the combined stimuli is usually at a maximum when the stimulus-interval is 4σ to 6σ.

Besides showing the existence of the enduring excitatory condition of c.e.s., the experiments on central summation also show that the c.e.s. which is produced in a motoneurone may be subliminal to varying degrees. Moreover, it can be concluded that a single centripetal impulse rarely, if ever, gives rise to a c.e.s. of more than subliminal value, for it is almost always[1] possible to make a stimulus so weak that it sets up several centripetal impulses, but yet fails to elicit a reflex response. That centripetal impulses are set up by such a stimulus is revealed by the resulting production of a subliminal grade of c.e.s. (recognizable as above by its power of summing with the other, also subliminal, c.e.s. produced by another centripetal volley). Therefore it follows that summation of the effects of several impulses is necessary to set up a reflex discharge. Both the repetitive nature of the discharge from receptor organs, and the great wealth of convergence paths in the central nervous system ensure that ample possibilities for central summation exist under normal conditions.

(b) When each centripetal volley produces a reflex response.

If both volleys are set up in the same afferent nerve and the second is made rather weaker than the first, all the impulses of the second volley will travel in fibres along which impulses of the first volley have already passed. When the interval between such volleys is short, the reflex contraction evoked by the second volley is due largely to the discharge of motoneurones which fail to respond to either volley alone [80]. The response of these motoneurones must have been due to a summation of the subliminal excitatory effects of each volley in the way described in the previous section.[2]

The question now arises: Why do not motoneurones, which

---

[1] The exceptional cases are probably due to the complicating effects of an ipselateral inhibition (p. 35).

[2] The method depends on the fact that one single maximal antidromic volley (pp. 38–9) in motor-nerve-fibres blocks one centrifugal impulse in each motor-nerve-fibre, so that only those centrifugal impulses discharged from a motoneurone after the first group can reach the muscle and evoke a contraction [79].

respond to the second volley alone, respond also when it is preceded by the first volley? This unresponsiveness which follows the first volley may persist for over 100 σ—sometimes for more than 400 σ [80, 93, 104], i.e. even when the second volley follows the first at these long intervals it evokes either no response or a response which is smaller than normal. Inhibition and refractory period are two possible causes of this unresponsiveness. The former effect could be due presumably to some of the impulses of the first volley being inhibitory in nature. The latter effect would follow the reflex response, and would be confined to those motoneurones which responded to the first volley.[1] Since the field of inhibition would not be restricted in this way, it is possible, under certain conditions, to distinguish between the effects of refractory period and inhibition. Thus, in those cases where unresponsiveness persists for more than 80 σ after the first volley, it can always be shown to be due to inhibition, for it is present both in the motoneurones which respond to the first volley and in those which do not. For example, if the first centripetal volley is so weak that it evokes a reflex discharge from very few motoneurones, it often greatly reduces the response evoked by a much more powerful second centripetal volley. In one observation the first centripetal volley produced a response of only 10 grm., but it reduced the response to a second centripetal volley from 240 grm. to 60 grm. when the interval between the two volleys was 50 σ [80]. It is clear that the stimulus setting up the first centripetal volley, although too weak to excite many excitatory fibres, excited many inhibitory fibres.

In cases where the response to the second volley has been reduced only when it follows the first at less than 30 σ, it has not yet been possible to show whether or not this reduction is due to inhibition.

Finally, in some cases the response to the second volley is not reduced even when the interval between the volleys is only 16 σ. At intervals shorter than this, the effect is masked by the response of additional motoneurones which are brought in by facilitation.

[1] It is important to realize that a refractory period always follows the reflex discharge of a motoneurone regardless of the simultaneous presence of inhibition.

(c) *The latent period of the response to the second of two centripetal volleys.*

When the interval between the two volleys in either the same nerve or different nerves is comparatively brief, the shortest latent period of the response to the second volley is less than normal [79]. Where the volleys are set up in different nerves, the response at any interval can be investigated without complication from the refractory period of the afferent pathway. In such cases the latent period of the second response is usually shortest at intervals of 6–8 σ. At longer intervals the latent period is less affected and at intervals of 20 σ or more it is usually unchanged. At briefer intervals also the latent period is less affected, and, when both volleys are set up simultaneously, it is seldom more than 1 σ shorter than normal [23, 29, 30, 31].

When both volleys are set up in the same afferent nerve, the effects are similar for intervals of 6 σ or longer, but with shorter intervals the effect of the refractory period of the nerve following the first volley is a complicating factor. The motoneurones which respond at these greatly reduced latent periods are, for the most part, those which are not excited by either volley alone. They are in the subliminal fringe of each volley, and their response is due to facilitation [69].

No part of the shortening of the latent period can be accounted for by reduction of the conduction time in the peripheral pathways. It must occur at the expense of the central reflex time. If the central reflex time is calculated by the method described (p. 19), it is found to be very short when the latent period of the second response is a minimum. Thus in two experiments it was 0·3 σ and 0·4 σ respectively, and in no experiment is it probably more than 1 σ. Now just as there can be no reduction in the peripheral conduction time, so there can be no reduction in the conduction time along central reflex pathways. Therefore it is concluded that, at least in some experiments, the central *conduction time* is normally not more than 0·5 σ. The remainder of the normal central reflex time is occupied at some central part of the reflex arc. There a nerve-impulse presumably gives rise to an excitatory condition which endures for some time before setting up an impulse in the next part of the central

pathway, i.e. there is delay at that point. This excitatory condition is undoubtedly the *c.e.s.* which has already been postulated to explain summation, and which is located most probably
at the synapses. Central *reflex time* is, therefore, the sum of
the central *conduction time* and the *synaptic delay*.

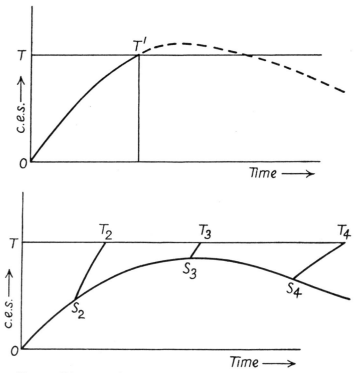

FIG. 15. Diagrammatic representation of the *c.e.s.* of a motoneurone
plotted as ordinates against time as abscissae.

All experimental observations on latent period can be satis-
factorily accounted for if it be assumed that, in any motoneurone,
the *c.e.s.* produced by a single centripetal volley gradually rises
to a maximum over a period of several sigmata and then slowly
declines as shown in Fig. 15 [79]. This is probably the result of a
temporal dispersion of the incident excitatory impulses, a condition indicated by other experimental observations (p. 41). On *Note* 18
the above assumption the 'synaptic delay' which normally occurs

will be the time necessary to build up *c.e.s.* to threshold value. Thus in Fig. 15, if OT is the threshold value of *c.e.s.*, TT^1 is the synaptic delay.

Note 19   The temporal dispersion of the reflex discharge is the result of differences in the 'synaptic' delays in the different motoneurones. The more intense the excitation of a motoneurone, the shorter the 'synaptic' delay is likely to be, and hence the shorter latent periods of stronger reflexes. Finally Fig. 15 shows how the shortening of the latent period of the second response can be explained. $OS_2S_3S_4$ represents the course of the subliminal *c.e.s.* produced in a motoneurone by the first centripetal volley. When the foremost impulses of the second centripetal volley are incident at S_3, it is clear that the 'synaptic' delay for that motoneurone (interval between S_3 and T_3) would be much shorter than for motoneurones which responded to a single volley, e.g. TT^1 in Fig. 15. In motoneurones where the *c.e.s.* just failed to reach threshold, the 'synaptic' delay would be so much shorter than S_3T_3 as to be negligible, and the central reflex time would be almost entirely a central conduction time. At shorter or longer intervals between the volleys the 'synaptic' delay would be longer than at S_3, e.g. at S_2 and S_4 in Fig. 15. The interval between the volleys at which there is the shortest 'synaptic' delay corresponds to the interval between the beginning of the *c.e.s.* production and the attainment of the maximum intensity in the average motoneurone. Values of 6σ to 8σ are usual for this interval in experiments where the centripetal volleys are set up in different afferent nerves.

Note 20   THE EFFECT OF AN ANTIDROMIC VOLLEY ON THE REFLEX
RESPONSE TO A SINGLE CENTRIPETAL VOLLEY [74]

When a single maximal (for the motor-fibres) break-shock is applied to the intact motor-nerve by electrodes *a* (Fig. 16), it sets up two volleys of impulses which travel in opposite directions. One, the centrifugal volley, passes to the muscle and excites it to respond by a maximal twitch, and the other, the centripetal, passes to the spinal cord. Since all the afferent nerve-fibres have been cut, the only centripetal impulses to reach the spinal cord will be in the motor-nerve-fibres (antidromic impulses). A maximal motor twitch is the muscular response evoked by a single maximal break-shock applied through electrodes a. (Therefore an antidromic volley does not evoke a discharge of nerve-impulses from motoneurones.) On the other hand, for some time after an antidromic volley has reached the motoneurones, it is more difficult to set up a reflex discharge [63, 74]. For example, the reflex response to a centripetal volley is reduced by an antidromic volley which precedes it by a short interval. If that interval be made shorter, all the reflex response is blocked, provided that there is no repetitive after-discharge (p. 42). Thus a single centripetal volley does not evoke a reflex discharge from motoneurones within $5\,\sigma$ of the arrival of an antidromic volley, but at about $10\cdot5\,\sigma$ after an antidromic volley the motoneurones have recovered their normal responsiveness.

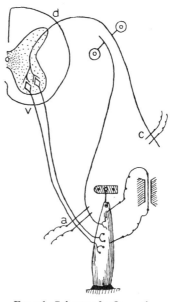

It has been concluded that this effect of an antidromic volley is due to the setting up of a refractory period in the motoneurones—at first absolute, later relative—having a

FIG. 16. Schema of reflex pathway and recording systems. v, ventral root. d, dorsal root. a, electrodes on uncut nerve to muscle. c, electrodes on afferent nerve.

total duration of about $10\cdot5\,\sigma$. Although the unresponsive period lasts for $5\,\sigma$ after an antidromic volley, this is not the duration of the absolute refractory period, because the effect of the centripetal volley cannot be made adequately strong, owing to the insufficiency of afferent terminals. The true absolute refractory period of the motoneurones is much shorter, for it is possible to set up two antidromic volleys, without hindrance from the absolute refractory period of nerve ($1\,\sigma$), at such a short interval that the second reaches the synapses of the motoneurones only $2 \cdot 5 \sigma$ after the first. The absolute refractory period of the motoneurones must, therefore, be less than $2 \cdot 5 \sigma$.

THE REFRACTORY PERIOD OF THE REFLEX ARC [26, 80]

The present view of the mechanism of setting up reflex discharges conceives of the refractory period of the arc being identical with the refractory period of the motoneurone after reflex discharge, although each particular part of the reflex arc has, of course, its own characteristic but shorter refractory period. The direct determination, however, of refractory period of the arc by observing the reflex responses to two centripetal volleys at various intervals apart is fraught with difficulties. For example, it is always difficult to distinguish between inhibition and refractory period as causes of unresponsiveness, while at short intervals facilitation brings about the response of additional motoneurones and so further complicates the picture. But in certain experiments where facilitation is brief and inhibition absent, it is possible to conclude that the total duration of the refractory period is not more than 16σ [80]. In other experiments, there may be a relative unresponsiveness for as long as 30σ, and this cannot be shown to be due to inhibition. Whether these cases are examples of a longer refractory period is uncertain.

By another and indirect method, using antidromic impulses in the motor-nerve, it is possible to arrive at values for the duration of the refractory period of the reflex arc. The refractory period following an antidromic impulse should be identical with that following a reflex discharge, for both travel over a similar path. The values which have been determined for the duration of the central refractory period following an antidromic impulse should, therefore, apply also to the central refractory period of the reflex arc. The value of $10 \cdot 5 \sigma$ arrived at by the indirect method [74] for the total duration of the refractory period is in agreement with the results obtained by the direct method which shows it to be shorter than 16σ. But the unresponsiveness which lasts as long as 30σ in that type of experiment receives no satisfactory explanation, and requires future investigation.

THE EFFECT OF AN ANTIDROMIC VOLLEY ON THE
CENTRAL EXCITATORY STATE

The subliminal excitatory state in the reflex centres produced by one centripetal volley is revealed by the facilitation of the response to a second centripetal volley following the first at a short interval. In order to investigate the effect of an antidromic volley on the *c.e.s.*, it must be timed so that it reaches the motoneurones after the production of *c.e.s.* by the first centripetal volley and before the arrival of the second centripetal volley. Under such circumstances the facilitation of the response to the second volley is greatly diminished in almost all cases [74]. This diminution cannot be explained by the refractory period set up by the antidromic volley, for the second response is diminished even when it follows the antidromic volley by an interval much longer than the duration of the refractory period. Therefore, when the antidromic volley reaches the motoneurones, it must inactivate some of the *c.e.s.* which has been set up by the first centripetal volley and which normally facilitates the response to the second volley. In all experiments a considerable inactivation of *c.e.s.* has been found. Some experiments are remarkable for the long duration of the *c.e.s.* produced by the first centripetal volley. When a long interval separates the two centripetal volleys in these experiments, the facilitation of the second volley is diminished only if the antidromic volley precedes it by a comparatively short interval. Now it seems likely from other observations that the impulses of the first centripetal volley do not reach the motoneurones synchronously, but suffer considerable temporal dispersion, e.g. from $5\,\sigma$ to $50\,\sigma$. In consequence, if the antidromic volley reaches the motoneurones too soon after the foremost impulses of the first centripetal volley, there will still be delayed impulses arriving after the antidromic volley, and the *c.e.s.* set up by them will facilitate the response to the second centripetal volley. If, however, the antidromic volley arrives after the delayed excitatory impulses there will be no facilitation. Thus these apparently exceptional cases can be explained by assuming temporal dispersion of excitatory impulses.

From histological considerations it is probable that an antidromic impulse, after passing up a motor-nerve-fibre and reaching a motoneurone, traverses the surface of the motoneurone including its dendrites and its further travel is limited only at the numerous synapses bordering on the perikaryon and dendrites. The inactivation of *c.e.s.* by an antidromic impulse therefore accords with the hypothesis that the formation of *c.e.s.* takes place at the synapses.

Note 21   AFTER-DISCHARGE

A moderately strong break-shock applied to an ipselateral afferent nerve evokes, in many preparations, a reflex discharge which continues for many sigmata [8, 10, 185, 186]. This prolonged discharge is called 'after-discharge'. It follows the initial reflex outburst and is due to the repeated responses of some motoneurones [185]. Therefore there must be a prolonged excitatory condition at some part of the central reflex pathway.

Knowledge of the nature of this central condition is gained by observing the effect of an antidromic volley on after-discharge [63, 81]. Following the antidromic volley, there is a complete block of all after-discharge for a period varying from $20\,\sigma$ to $60\,\sigma$ according to the intensity of the after-discharge, e.g. Fig. 17. A block of similar duration has also been found for the after-discharge which follows a tetanic flexor reflex. This period of 20–$60\,\sigma$ is too long to be due to the refractory period set up by the antidromic volley, for that is only about $10\cdot5\,\sigma$ in duration [74]. The inactivation of *c.e.s.* must be the cause of the long period of quiescence. The re-commencement of after-discharge following this period parallels the building-up of fresh *c.e.s.* after the inactivation of preformed *c.e.s.* by an antidromic volley. Therefore the reappearance of the after-discharge probably is due to the temporal dispersion of the excitatory impulses.

The question now arises: Is all the after-discharge which normally occurs to be attributed to such delayed excitatory impulses? When a motoneurone discharges a centrifugal impulse, i.e. a reflex discharge, this impulse must traverse the same path as the antidromic impulse, but the direction of travel, for the most part, would be the reverse. If, as seems probable, the effect of the propagated disturbance on any part of the motoneurone does not depend on the direction of its travel, the

effect of a reflex discharge on a motoneurone should be indistinguishable from the effect of an antidromic impulse. It has
already been concluded that an antidromic volley inactivates
preformed *c.e.s.*, and so it is probable that a reflex discharge is
also associated with a considerable inactivation of the *c.e.s.* of

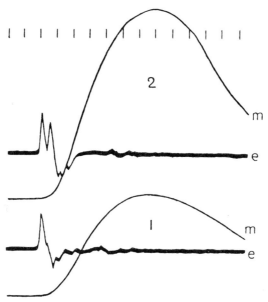

FIG. 17. Electrical *e* and mechanical *m* records of responses of tibialis
anticus muscle set up as follows:
(1) By a single break-shock to the posterior tibial nerve.
(2) By a single break-shock to the posterior tibial nerve followed 19·8 σ
later by a single break-shock to the intact motor-nerve (peroneal).
Time, 10 σ.

a motoneurone. Following that inactivation the *c.e.s.* has to be
built up to threshold value before another discharge can occur.
If this is so, repeated discharges of a motoneurone, i.e. after-
discharge, can only occur when the formation of *c.e.s.* continues
to take place, and this in turn must be due to the continued
arrival of excitatory impulses. The 'delay paths' postulated by
Forbes [89] are the probable source of the continuous bombardment of a motoneurone by excitatory impulses originating in a
single centripetal volley. The delay may arise partly in the peri-

pheral pathway owing to some fibres conducting impulses at a faster rate than others, and partly in the spinal cord owing to delay at the synapses of internuncial neurones, and to the conduction time in some central paths being longer than in others [87]. Normally the after-discharges of individual motoneurones are out-of-phase with one another—hence the almost uninterrupted sequence of small action-currents in the electrical response. If an antidromic volley affects each motoneurone exactly as if a reflex discharge had taken place, the result is equivalent to a momentary synchronization of the after-discharges of all the motoneurones, and there follows the quiescent period during which no after-discharge occurs. The duration of this period must be similar to the interval between the successive discharges of those motoneurones whose after-discharge has the most rapid rhythm so that the duration of the quiescent period affords a measure of the most rapid rhythm of afterdischarge. Rhythms of 20 to 50 per sec. are most commonly observed.

Since the interval between two successive discharges of a motoneurone is the time taken in building up c.e.s. to threshold value, the frequency of rhythm of after-discharge at any instant is conditioned by the rate at which c.e.s. is being built up in that motoneurone. The interval between successive discharges is almost always longer than $10 \cdot 5 \sigma$, which is the duration of the refractory period of a motoneurone, and so the recovery period of the excitability of a motoneurone after its discharge usually does not influence the interval before its next discharge. The rhythm of after-discharge of a motoneurone is conditioned by the rate of building-up of c.e.s. from excitatory impulses and not by the rate of recovery from its refractory period.

It is to be noted that the present conceptions indicate that it is not possible to have a c.e.s. of supraliminal value, for, as soon as threshold is reached, a discharge will be set up with consequent disappearance of c.e.s.

THE NATURE OF THE CENTRAL EXCITATORY STATE

Central summation of excitatory effects is an experimental fact, and the term 'central excitatory state' has been used so far as a name for an enduring central excitatory process without any implications as to its nature. There are some differences of opinion about the nature of *c.e.s.* The extreme views are perhaps represented as follows:

1. That the electrical responses of successive nerve-impulses summate, on analogy with the 'retention of action-current' of crustacean nerve, or the negative after-potential of vertebrate nerve [94].

2. That each nerve-impulse produces a quantum of exciting agent, a chemical substance, which sums with other quanta formed at the same or neighbouring points by other impulses [95]. The disappearance of *c.e.s.* after an antidromic impulse shows that *c.e.s.* must at least be largely restricted to those parts of the motoneurone which are accessible to such an impulse, i.e. to the surface membrane of the perikaryon and dendrites, for, in analogy to peripheral nerve, the impulse should traverse the surface membrane of the motoneurone. It does not seem possible that a chemical substance, such as is postulated in the second hypothesis, would be restricted to the surface membrane of the motoneurone or be inactivated by an antidromic impulse.

In criticism of the first hypothesis it may be pointed out that the negative after-potential of vertebrate nerve is possibly an abnormal condition of excised peripheral nerve resulting from absence of blood-supply and fatigue, as is shown by its close relation to the supernormal phase [103]. Again, it is improbable that an antidromic impulse would diminish negative after-potential, but rather that it would add to the existing negative after-potential. There is another process in peripheral nerve which may give a clue to the nature of *c.e.s.*, namely the local excitatory state [32, 124]. It is an excitatory process localized to the stimulated region of the excitable tissue, and it is capable of summation. Although very short in duration in peripheral nerve (about 1 σ at most), it is longer in other excitable tissues, e.g. it has a duration of at least 8 σ in heart-muscle. Moreover, the removal of local excitatory state at a point by the passage of a nerve-impulse is analogous to the disappearance of *c.e.s.* after an antidromic volley or a reflex discharge. Thus it seems likely the *c.e.s.* is a specialized manifestation of the local excitatory state [82, 186]. According to the membrane theory [19, 123] of nerve conduction the local excitatory state is a partial depolarization of the membrane surrounding the axis cylinders of nerve-fibres. By analogy, *c.e.s.* is probably a depolarization of those parts of the surface membranes of motoneurones on which excitatory impulses impinge, i.e. the synaptic membranes. It has been stated that some summation of the *c.e.s.* is produced by excitatory impulses reaching different synapses of the same motoneurone. The mechanism of this summation is not clear, but it must be remembered that the surface membrane of the motoneurone is common to all its synapses, so that a change at any one synapse, e.g. due to the formation of *c.e.s.*, could be accompanied by changes at other synapses.

Note 22

Note 23

IV

THE STRETCH REFLEX

[184]

IF the tendon of a healthy muscle is drawn upon by an antagonistic muscle or by the manipulations of the investigator or by the movement of a joint in response to gravity, the muscle actively resists the extending force. A muscle which has been paralysed by section of its motor-nerve or of the ventral or dorsal roots supplying it, does not actively resist and behaves like a piece of non-contractile tissue such as skin. The muscle is flaccid. The resistance, however, from a muscle in full connexion with the nervous system is a reflex contraction, 'the stretch reflex'.[1] The special feature of the reflex is that impulses from tension receptors within the muscle itself cause its development (proprioceptive reflex). In the unstretched muscle no centripetal impulses are set up by the tension receptors. An extending force to the tendon stretches the muscle and excites a discharge of impulses from the tension receptors. The frequency of discharge from a single receptor organ may be as high as 250 impulses a second [131].

It is probable that all tension receptors are not affected simultaneously by a small pull, but that increase of pull adds to the number of end-organs involved—'recruitment' at the periphery. As the pull progresses, those organs first affected become most affected and respond with the highest frequencies of discharge, while those which are more lately recruited respond with lower frequencies.

Thus it comes about that as the tendon is pulled upon from a position of rest, the numerous tension receptors are recruited one after another and, each at different frequencies, send nerve-impulses through the dorsal roots of the spinal cord to those motoneurones which supply the muscle-fibres of this selfsame muscle. If only a few receptors are made active by the pull on the tendon, only a few motoneurones are excited to discharge. If more receptors are affected, as by a stronger pull on the

---

[1] Or myotatic reflex = μῦς, muscle: τάτος, extended.

tendon, more motoneurones are excited and more muscle-fibres are activated in opposition to the increased pull. Thus the number of muscle-fibres responding to the pull is automatically regulated and controlled, *pari passu*, by the degree of tension on the tendon.

The nature of the reflex response was first shown in the de-cerebrated animal. The exaggeration of postural 'tone' in this

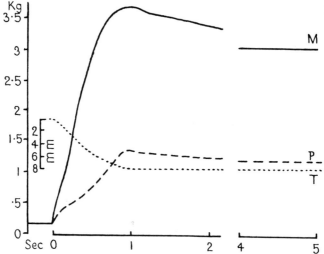

FIG. 18. Whole quadriceps. Muscular response *M* before, and after *P* cutting nerve to muscle, to stretch of 8 mm. *T* indicator of table-fall. Time in secs. Scales at side show (i) tension on the tendon, (ii) distance of table's descent in mm.

preparation makes it especially favourable for observation [119]. The tendon of the vasto-crureus muscle was attached to a rigidly held but delicate isometric myograph. All other muscles in that and the other leg had been paralysed by section of their nerves and the skin was also denervated or protected from extraneous stimuli. Underneath the myograph and separate from it was a table to which the femur was held by steel drills and on which the trunk of the preparation lay. The top of the table could be moved up and down under the myograph so as to slacken or pull on the tendon. The descent of the table-top was operated by an hydraulic plunger whose rate was easily controlled. The rates and extent of the descent corresponded with natural movements of the knee-joint. When the table descended, the myograph traced a convex curve, i.e. the increment of tension per mm. fall of the table-top became less as the extent of the stretch increased (Fig. 18). This convexity alone suggested some tension added by reflex action over and above that produced by the dead stretch of the tendon and muscle. The exact amount of the reflexly added tension was seen when the muscle was paralysed by cutting its nerve and the table-top was allowed to descend once again and pull on the tendon. The tension in the myogram was much less and the curve concave.

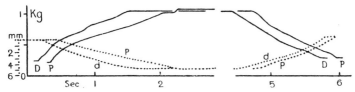

FIG. 19. Whole quadriceps, deafferented 112 days. Comparison of deafferented *D* and paralytic *P* (by nerve section) muscle to two comparable 5 mm. stretches, *d* applied to deafferented muscle, *p* to paralysed muscle. Time in secs.

This concave curve is the tension-curve of a denervated or excised muscle and is the response of passive muscle. If centripetal impulses from the tendon organs are interrupted by section of the dorsal spinal roots ('deafferentation'), the behaviour of the muscle resembles that of an excised muscle (Fig. 19).[1] Again, activity of the reflex centres of the muscle is prevented by stimulation of any nerve which evokes the flexor reflex in that limb, i.e. if the centres are inhibited, traction on the tendon evokes only a passive response—the reflex contraction is abolished (Fig. 20). This last method has the advantage of not doing irreparable damage like section of the motor-nerve or dorsal roots, and can be repeated time and again.

When the knee of an intact animal is straightened and the leg extended, the tendons of the flexor muscles in the thigh are

[1] This is certainly true so far as response to stretch is concerned. Nevertheless, the muscles of some preparations do show phasic or maintained contraction after section of the dorsal roots. In these cases, the exciting impulses come from higher centres, e.g. labyrinth, thalamus, or cerebral cortex, or travel by other and intact afferent nerves from the periphery of the body to the motor centres.

drawn upon and the flexor muscles are lengthened. So when the stretch reflex of the knee-extensor is elicited in a prepared animal, and the tendons of antagonistic flexor muscles are drawn upon during this time, the stretch reflex is inhibited, often completely (Fig. 21; cf. Fig. 36, p. 71). This method of inhibition is beyond criticism which can be levelled at wholesale electrical stimulation of fibres of different function in a cutaneous or mixed nerve [120].

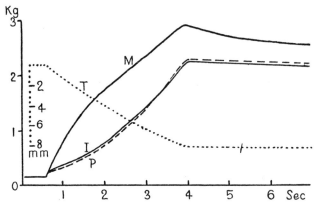

FIG. 20. Rectus femoris 8 mm. stretch *T*. Reaction of uninhibited muscle *M*, of reflexly inhibited muscle *I*, and of paralysed (by nerve section) muscle *P* (broken line). The inhibition began before and continued during the whole record. *T* indicator of table fall.

When the tendon of a muscle is drawn upon very suddenly as, for instance, by a tap at some point where it is not supported by underlying bone, e.g. the patellar tendon as it passes over the knee-joint or the tendo Achillis at the ankle, a number of tension receptors are subjected to a sudden brief stretch, so that they send to the cord an almost synchronous volley of nerve-impulses, which, by summation of central effect *c.e.s.*, excite a number of Note 24 motoneurones to discharge. The outcome is a tendon-jerk of which the knee-jerk is the most familiar example (Fig. 22). Tendon-jerks are regarded as the 'phasic reaction' of the stretch reflex, whereas the slower and longer continued pull of the tendon evokes, by continued excitation from the same reflex path, the 'static reaction' of the stretch reflex.

The smallest stretch of a tendon which is adequate to elicit a tendon-jerk is not known accurately but, in a muscle of which the fibres have an average length of 40 mm., a sudden incremental stretch from a tap of less than 10μ evokes a jerk [66].[1] The latent period of the stretch organ in the muscle in response to a sudden increment of stretch is very brief, probably about $1-2\,\sigma$. The latent period of the stretch reflex, as such, in response to a slow increment, has only an artificial interest since, as explained above, the rate of stretching determines the rate of discharge from individual organs and the degree of stretching determines the number of organs excited. The latent period of the knee-jerk is so short that for many years there was some doubt about

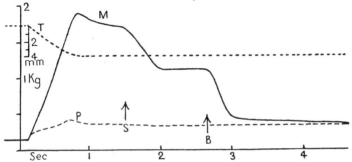

FIG. 21. Response of quadriceps to stretch T of 4 mm., before M, and after P severance of its nerve. During the response M, a stretch of semitendinosus begins approximately at S, followed by a stretch of biceps at B.

its being a reflex [111]. Even now that the demur has been shown Note 25 to be groundless, the rate of conduction of nerve-impulses being much higher than was then thought, e.g. as high as 80 metres a second,[2] it is still evident that the pathway in the cord must be direct and the passage very brief. While the tendon-jerk is one of the last to disappear in anaesthesia and circulatory collapse, the static stretch reflex fails much sooner. The reason for this is not altogether clear. The difference may be due to less intense (because more asynchronous) summation at the synapses in the static reflex.

[1] This figure may be compared with the smallness of movements at joints which is perceived by consciousness (Goldscheider [162]).
[2] 60–90 metres a second in efferent [20, 84, 85, 87], probably at least 50 metres a second in afferent fibres.

The nervous arc in this reflex is short, as explained above. The path through the cord is confined to a small number of segments, for the efferent fibres of the muscles are segmentally similar to the afferent fibres. Both the *phasic* and *static* reactions can be elicited from leg muscles when the lumbar region of the cord has been isolated from the midbrain and higher centres. The phasic reaction (knee-jerk) is more resistant to interference, for it can be elicited from one of the lower types of laboratory animal, such as the dog or cat, within a few minutes or even moments after the severance of the cord from higher centres. In many species of monkeys the jerk commonly does not return for several hours or days, although rarely it does not disappear at all. In man, slight evidence of the jerk can be detected after two or three weeks [101, 108, 147]. Even in the lower animals, however, the postural reaction is absent for a much longer time, as evidenced by the limpness and flaccidity of the hind-quarters which is the cardinal sign in the condition of 'spinal shock'. In the dog, after two or three weeks, the shock passes off and the muscles reacquire resistance to stretch. That is, the stretch reflex returns and, with lapse of time, becomes quite evident, at least at the ankle. At length, the limb becomes stiff from 'hypertonia' of the extensor muscles. Their state comes to resemble that ensuing when the brain-stem has been divided in the quadrigeminal region, 'decerebrate rigidity' [67].

Action-currents of muscles in the stretch reflex.

It is not difficult to examine the action-currents of muscles, and in man they can be observed by plunging a small hypodermic needle with an insulated core through the skin into the muscle [10]. Such an electrode leads off the action-currents from a restricted group of muscle-fibres. If at first the muscle is at absolute rest there will be no action-currents. On passive extension of the muscle whereby the stretch reflex is elicited, small action-currents begin at a rate of 10–25 per sec.

Lower figures, e.g. 7–20, represent the actual rate of firing of the motor units engaged at that particular tension, while higher rates, e.g. 20–25, need not be due entirely to an *actual* increase of rate of firing of each unit but partly to asynchronism between different units giving rise to an *apparent* increase in rate. But as the tension on the tendon increases, the actual rate of discharge of any given unit increases, and at the same time, owing to peripheral recruitment of tension receptors asynchronism comes more into evidence, so that eventually *apparent* rates of 200–250 per sec. can be recorded, although the actual rate of any one unit is even then much slower, e.g. 30–40.

This experiment has its counterpart in the laboratory animal when a muscle showing decerebrate rigidity is slightly extended. The familiar small irregular action-currents appear [43, 72]. When the extension is increased, either in the human subject or in the preparation, the number of vibrations increases, but the striking change is an increase in the summed potential of the action-currents, since many more units are recruited into the reflex and each fresh unit adds its quota of action-current (Fig. 24). This summing of action-current potential continues as long as the muscle is extended. The action-currents, therefore, of natural muscular movements, whether voluntary or proprioceptive, show as irregular oscillations, provided that the recording instrument is recording from a number of fibres. The oscillations are irregular because the muscle-fibres contract asynchronously. The amplitude of the vibrations is some guide to the number of muscle-fibres which are active, but because of their asynchronism they are an unreliable guide to the rate of discharge of spinal centres. 'Voluntary contraction in man is maintained by a series of nerve-impulses which range from 5 to 50 or more per sec. in each nerve-fibre.' When the cerebral motor cortex is stimulated artificially, the discharge can then be driven to a rate as high as 120 per sec. [54].

In the stretch reflex asynchronism is much in evidence, especially if silver pins are used in the experiment, for these being conductors throughout their length lead off action-currents from all the fibres with which they are in contact. But the asynchronism can be reduced by diminishing the number of motor units. This is achieved by cutting some of the ventral spinal roots. If this is cautiously continued, step by step, in the final stage the string gives small discrete regular vibrations about 7–20 times per sec. when the stretch on the tendon is slight [10, 63]. This is the rate of discharge of a single motoneurone. So long as the tension on the tendon is slight,

E

such a muscle as M. soleus in the cat shows this rate even if more than one motoneurone has been spared in the root section. But if the tension be increased a little, another unit may be brought into action, perhaps at some rate like 8 or 9 per sec. A double series of action-currents registers this change and the individual waves of each series pass and repass one another (Fig. 25). Even without section of ventral roots, M. soleus of the cat is a favourable muscle for observing the rate of discharge of single motoneurones [63]. When the tendon is slightly drawn upon, the only activity may be the discharge of a single motoneurone, 7–8 times per sec. On drawing the tendon somewhat farther, more motoneurones are recruited and within 0·05 sec. the record shows again the small irregular vibrations. With relaxation of the tendon, the irregular rhythm subsides until three, two, and finally one regular series of waves is visible.

The sum total of spinal discharge in a stretched muscle is asynchronous because the centripetal impulses are already asynchronous before they reach the centre and so the centrifugal impulses are, *a fortiori*, more asynchronous.

If a single unit in a decerebrated preparation is firing at a certain rate, hastening or slowing of the discharge can be brought about by altering the position of the head. We see here, in fact, an elemental aspect of the control of posture by the reflexes from the labyrinth and neck muscles. With the snout turned toward the side to which the muscle belongs, the rate of discharge is increased by this 'maximum' position. When the snout is turned away from the muscle, the rate is diminished— minimum position [65].

Lengthening and shortening reactions in postural muscle.

If an attempt be made to bend the knee or ankle of a decerebrated animal or of an animal with an isolated spinal cord ('chronic spinal' animal), one's hand meets resistance from those muscles which extend the joint. The attempt is, in fact, causing a further accentuation of the stretch reflex in muscles which are *Note 26* already highly responsive to stretching. If the attempt to flex the joint is maintained, there comes a point and time at which the muscle suddenly gives way and allows any degree of flexion to be imposed upon it ('clasp-knife' effect). This is the 'lengthening reaction' [177], and it marks the partial or total abolition of the stretch reflex. If the knee-extensor, vasto-crureus, be subjected to an extension of 3 mm., i.e. about 2 per cent. increase in length, the stretch reflex so elicited maintains itself unchanged for half an hour or longer. But if the extension is 7 mm., the stretch reflex will then subside entirely in five or ten minutes. The nervous mechanism concerned may well be operated by the cumulative inhibitory effect from the strong motor discharge. The course of events is probably as follows. One must suppose that the centres receive impulses from the tension receptors and they respond by evoking the stretch reflex. During the stretch reflex, however, certain other end-organs send inhibitory impulses to the centre but they are relatively infrequent and asynchronous, in contrast to the excitatory. The central excitatory state, therefore, is not diminished perceptibly until a stage when the tension is considerable and possibly dangerous. At that stage the inhibitory impulses gain ascendancy and the muscle relaxes. Now any inhibition of the reflex centre of the extensor muscle in one leg has its counterpart in excitation of the extensor muscle of the other leg (Principle of Reciprocal Innervation). With autogenetic inhibition of the forcibly flexed knee-extensor (the 'lengthening reaction') there ensues excitation of the opposite knee-extensor. This latter is Philippson's reflex [137, 177].

A muscle which shows the lengthening reaction shows also the shortening reaction [177]. Thus, if the ends of the muscle are approximated, the muscle is slackened, but only momentarily, for it quickly adjusts its length and 'stays put', so holding the limb at the angle imposed, by developing a sufficient static tension. It seems probable that here the relief of tension during the execution of the 'shortening' lessens the autogenous reflex excitation for the time being, but this sets in again on cessation of that relief.

Activity of the stretch organ. Autogenetic inhibition.

The electrogram of a muscle during elicitation of the tendon-jerk reveals a large single deviation which in actual time just precedes the upstroke of the myogram (Fig. 22). When this has subsided, the electrogram becomes absolutely motionless for a considerable period during which the myogram attains its plateau and begins to subside [62, 98]. During the subsidence, rapid movements begin again in the electrogram. The cause of *Note* 27 this 'silent period' in the electrogram was believed at one time to be due entirely to reflex inhibition from some inhibitory organ within the muscle. It has been shown, however, with a peripheral nerve-muscle preparation in the frog that, during the rising phase of a muscle twitch, there is cessation of electrical discharge which is believed to be due to slackening the strain of tendon-pull on the non-contracting muscle-spindle [98, 132]. This cessation continues as long as the spindle is relieved of strain. Fig. 23 shows the effect in a mammalian tension receptor.

When frog's muscle is strongly excited, so that the intrafusal fibres themselves contract as well as the ordinary muscle-fibres, the spindle is under strain throughout the process and discharges all the time without the supervention of a silent period [132].

It is therefore unnecessary to postulate any but a peripheral mechanism for the silent period.

Although the silent period itself need not be due to inhibition, there is good evidence of inhibition in and from a muscle in reflex activity during a single-volley reflex like a tendon-jerk. The muscle itself in the knee-jerk (vasto-crureus) shows a silent period, but at the same time distant muscles like gastrocnemius have also in their electrogram a silent period which is certainly reflex in origin [62]. Moreover, when the tendon of soleus (extensor) is tapped, the tibialis anticus (flexor) receives a reflex excitatory volley during the silent period of the soleus jerk.

One may conclude, therefore, that reflex inhibition occurs during the silent period.[1] Other extensors are thereby inhibited while flexors are excited, in accordance with the Principle of Reciprocal Innervation.

The lengthening reaction has already been cited as evidence for autogenetic inhibition.

[1] The 'central refractory period', to give the phenomenon an earlier name [63], must overlap with the silent period of a reflex like the knee-jerk.

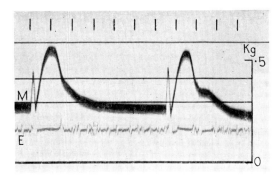

FIG. 22. M. Gastrocnemius. Decerebrate preparation. Two tendon-jerks during slight reflex. Taps on tendon show as sharp peaks in myogram. Note well marked hump in second jerk. In the electrogram, the 'silent period' after the jerk is to be compared with FIG. 23. Time, 0·1 sec.

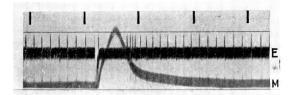

FIG. 23. Pause in electrical response (E) of one stretch receptor, in Peroneus longus of cat, during a motor twitch. Recorded with amplifier and oscillograph from electrodes on nerve just above a cut which severed all sensory fibres but one. (M.) Myograph record, initial tension 30 grms. Time, 0·1 sec.

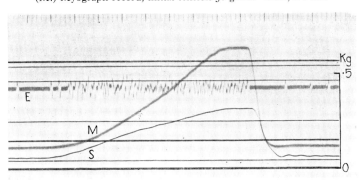

FIG. 24. M. Soleus. Decerebrate preparation. Stretch reflex from gradual lengthening of muscle (thin unsteady line S, rise of stretch indicator), followed by sudden release. Time, small divisions, 20 σ. Note in electrical record the discrete firing of units before and after the stretch, and the asynchronous confusion of firing during the stretch reflex. Immediately after the release the firing misses a beat.

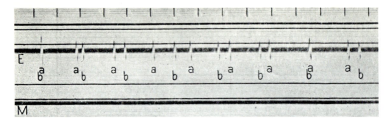

FIG. 25. M. Soleus. Decerebrate preparation. There is a small steady stretch in the muscle. One unit (*a*) fires 7 times a second, another unit (*b*) fires 5 to 5·5 times a second. Time, 0·1 sec.

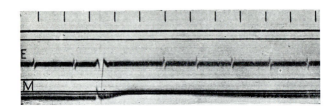

FIG. 27. M. Soleus. Decerebrate preparation. One unit in rhythmic discharge and interrupted by a light tendon-tap (sharp mechanical deflection) which causes a tendon-jerk. Following the large wave of the jerk (a single wave in many units) the original unit, after a silent period, begins beating at an accelerated rate which is maintained until the end of the plate. Time, 0·1 sec.

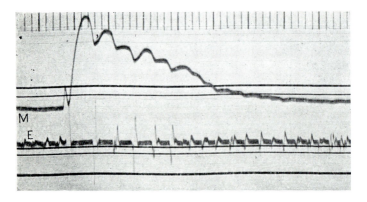

FIG. 30. M. Quadriceps. Decerebrate preparation. A slight stretch, previously applied, produces an obscured clonus. It is less obscured in the electrogram than in the myogram. A tendon-jerk is then elicited after which there follows a well-defined clonic after-discharge. Time, 20 σ.

'Red' and 'white' muscle [64].

In a laboratory animal like the rabbit or cat, the naked eye readily distinguishes two kinds of muscle—'red' and 'white'. This difference has long excited speculation. Early histologists noted these variations and observed that, in the rabbit, they could be correlated with differences in contraction. Some muscles of the rabbit such as soleus, semitendinosus and crureus are brick-red in colour, while most of the others are colourless and translucent. Ranvier showed that the red muscles contract more slowly than pale, and differ microscopically in being composed of granular fibres with more sarcoplasm and a marked longitudinal striation. Grützner, finding that the muscles of higher animals were composed of a mixture of granular and non-granular fibres, considered that these two types were intermingled in each muscle with a corresponding combination of function. It is now known, however, that the muscles of the cat, dog, and monkey are separable into two groups, as in the rabbit. The two groups in these animals still retain differences in the speed of contraction, although the difference in colour is only slight in the cat and dog, and evident only as a slightly dusky shade in man and the monkey. Furthermore, in all kinds of animals there is a general difference between the histological appearance of the slowly contracting fibres and the rapid fibres, namely that all slowly contracting fibres can store lipoid in the form of liposomes and become granular in appearance, while few rapid fibres have this property. In an emaciated animal all histological differences disappear, but the differences in contraction remain. Of the macroscopic criteria, opacity disappears with emaciation.

Red pigmentation is not inseparably connected with slow contraction, for it is found sometimes without corresponding slowness, e.g. pectoralis of the pigeon, and it may be absent from some slow muscles in higher mammals. Redness of muscles, when it occurs as in the cat, develops at a later stage of growth than the speed differences. There is, therefore, no absolute histological criterion of the speed of contraction of mammalian muscle.

It may be convenient to summarize the characteristics of muscle [64]:

	'Slow' muscle. *'Red.'*	*'Rapid' muscle.* *'Pale.'*
Myogram	Slow contraction and relaxation, e.g. 100–120 σ to the summit of the motor twitch (cat)	Rapid contraction and relaxation, e.g. 30–40 σ to the summit of the motor twitch (cat)
Electrogram	Slow action-current	Quick action-current
Colour when washed free of blood	Opaque red in rabbit, cat, and dog. Opaque and darker in fish and monkey. Opaque red in man	Translucent and colourless in rabbit, fish, and monkey. Less opaque red in cat and dog. Opaque red in man
Unstained fibre in cross-section (parallel, but less marked differences with ordinary stains)	Opaque and large in normal mammalia. Opaque and small in fish (ray)	Clear and smaller average size in rabbit. A mixture of clear and opaque fibres of sizes averaging the same as slow muscles in cat, dog, monkey, and man. Clear and large in fish (ray)
After staining with Sudan III or Scharlach R	In both types, opacity seen to be due to granules of lipoid nature	
Variation with nutrition	Every fibre has stored liposomes in a fat animal. Every fibre has become large in a large animal. Fibres clear in emaciation	A very few fibres can become loaded with liposomes, but these fibres do not become large. Most fibres can vary in size, but do not store liposomes. Fibres clear in emaciation
Sarcoplasm	Abundant in rabbit and bat	More scanty in rabbit. Abundant in fish and the rapid muscles of some insects

As a general rule the chief extensor muscles of all mammals possess a deep, slowly contracting component and a superficial rapid component, for example, soleus (slow) and gastrocnemius (rapid) in the ankle-extensors, crureus (slow) and vastus lateralis (rapid) in the knee-extensors, the medial short head of triceps (slow) and the lateral short head of triceps (rapid) in the elbow-extensor, and the deep head of supraspinatus (slow) and the superficial head (rapid) in the shoulder-extensor. Fibres of approximately equal contraction speed are thus collected as separate muscles, or 'heads' in the terminology of the anatomist. The flexor muscles as a rule are of the rapidly contracting variety. (Semitendinosus of the rabbit, the classical slow muscle of Ranvier, is really semimembranosus, a knee- and hip-extensor. In the dog, there is no muscle distinguishable anatomically as soleus.)

Early investigators postulated a dual mechanism for muscular contraction, slowly contracting muscles for tonic sustained con-

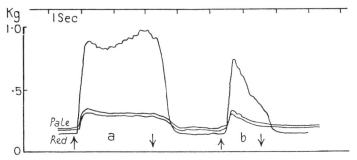

FIG. 26. The reflex effect of the labyrinthine and neck reflexes on red and pale muscle. Preparation with section of brain-stem slightly anterior to superior colliculi. M. triceps, short lateral head (pale), doubly-traced line, short medial head (red), single line. Neck dorsiflexed at ↑ and ventriflexed at ↓. Labyrinth in intermediate position in each neck posture.

traction and rapidly contracting muscles for phasic contractions. Recent investigations [63] have shown that there is a certain degree of truth in this hypothesis, for the slower muscles are, in fact, those in which the stretch reflex is most easily provoked and as will be seen later, the rapidly contracting muscles are those which take the earliest and greatest part in reflexes which involve rapid contraction. The greater readiness of slow muscles to respond to stretch is seen often in acute spinal transection, for they respond then, when the white component is in complete abeyance. Since the labyrinthine and neck reflexes exert their effect mainly upon the stretch reflex, it is not surprising to find 'red' muscle is distinguished for its readier response to the control from the labyrinth and neck, the latent period of 'red' muscle being less and its tension greater than that of 'white' muscle (Fig. 26).

Red muscles, therefore, contain the focus of the stretch reflex, a bulk of effectors of low threshold, while pale muscles contain stretch-reflex effectors of medium and high threshold and are devoted rather to kinetic reflexes. But both types of muscle are potentially involved in all reflexes and the difference between them is only relative, expressed in terms of threshold of spinal excitation [17, 36, 62, 64, 65, 99, 140].

In view of the fact that in the newborn animal all muscles are slow in contraction and that in the course of development the rapid muscles gradually acquire a greater speed in the whole contraction process [64], it would seem logical to suppose that the existence of these two types depends simply on differentiation of speed in contraction in those muscles which take most part in rapid reflexes where economy of energy is not a considerable factor.

'Rebound' in the stretch reflex.

When an inhibitory stimulus is applied by a single break-shock or otherwise, the discharge of a single motor unit is brought to a temporary standstill and is then accelerated. This acceleration of the discharge of impulses is a simple expression of 'rebound'. After it, the normal rate is resumed [63] (Fig. 27).[1]

The rebound is very striking after the silent period which follows a tendon-jerk [62], where the elevation in the myogram may be so evident as to deserve the name of 'hump' (Fig. 28).

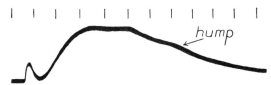

FIG. 28. Vasto-crureus in decerebrate preparation. Time, 0·2 sec.

In a perfectly quiescent preparation in which the continuous pull on the tendon is so slight that no units discharge, rebound after a tap may show itself as a transient outburst from one or two units.

---

[1] The relation of acceleration of tension organ discharge (Fig. 23) to reflex acceleration has not yet been examined.

Clonus.

When the stretch reflex is elicited in a favourable decerebrate preparation, it sometimes happens that the discharge of the motor units loses its asynchronous character and becomes synchronous. This synchronism may be initiated by a tap on the tendon, after which the volleys get 'into step' when the silent period is over and so continue. The myogram is then no longer smooth but shows an unfused series of small waves at regular intervals. This tremor in the muscle is 'clonus' (Fig. 29) [203]. We have given reasons for believing that the silent period, although not itself entirely an inhibition, may be contemporaneous with a

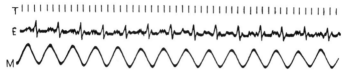

FIG. 29. Clonic response of quadriceps at 13 a second, elicited by attaching the muscle to an isotonic lever weighted by 1 kg. Time, 0·02 sec.

period of central inhibition. After any inhibition, rebound may occur. Here, the rebound contraction is the 'hump', which, when favoured by experimental conditions, is so exaggerated that it becomes as large as the jerk which gave it origin (Fig. 30). The continued rebound is clonus. Each wavelet of contraction is a rebound from a preceding inhibition or an excitation breaking through an inhibition, and so clonus represents a series of jerks evolved by the continued activity of an alternately self-exciting and self-inhibiting mechanism [63].

The effect of the sympathetic system.

The sympathetic nerve-supply to muscles is very slender. Whatever the function of that supply may be, it is not essentially concerned with the stretch reflex, at any rate, in cats and dogs, for cutting, degeneration, or stimulation of the sympathetic nerve to the muscle fail to produce qualitative change in the stretch reflex [63]. Some investigators believe that the sympathetic prevents peripheral fatigue [46, 114, 129, 134, 146]. After removal of the sympathetic in cats, there appears to be a change in the responsiveness of proprioceptive organs, possibly from vascular alterations [138, 139], and quantitative changes ensue in the reflex.

Blood-supply in postural muscle.

The stretch reflex provides clear evidence of agreement with the rule that capillaries in active muscle are dilated. Only a modest amount of pull on the tendon of a 'red' muscle will open up numerous capillaries and hasten the flow of blood in all of them to a remarkable extent. The phenomenon can easily be observed on the surface of M. soleus by using a low-power microscope and oblique illumination of the surface of the muscle [63]. Thus postural muscle receives an adequate supply of blood for the performance of its function.

V

REFLEXES IN EXTENSOR MUSCLES OTHER THAN POSTURAL REFLEXES

1. THE REFLEX OF CROSSED EXTENSION [117, 118, 140]

In myographic examination (Fig. 31) the characteristics of activity are

(i) long and variable latent period;

(ii) slow increase in tension. The rise to the plateau is often in two steps, i.e. sigmoid;

(iii) long after-discharge and slow decline.

i. The length of the latent period accords with the ensuing features. One single stimulus indeed may not be sufficient by itself to evoke a reflex. Only after repeating the stimulus does the reflex begin. Two distinct processes are concerned in this delay. The first is inevitable and characteristic of any transmission of physiological excitation—the conduction time. The second process occupies the summation period, which is due to synaptic delay through at least two series of synapses. During it, by the repetition of stimuli, the central excitatory state is raised from subliminal to liminal value. In this reflex, summation ('addition latente' [24, 115, 189]) is well marked and is typical. Its duration is extremely variable. This inertia in the march of events originates in the reflex centres, for direct stimulation of the motor-nerve throws the muscle into contraction (Fig. 32) which differs only in small respects from the motor response of a flexor muscle (Fig. 10, a).

So from the outset it is clear that the reflex centres impose greater modification on the response in the crossed extensor reflex than in the flexor reflex. It is believed that an internuncial neurone is always involved.

ii. Even when elicited, the reflex develops its sigmoid ascent so gradually that a period may elapse ten to twenty times longer than in the motor-nerve tetanus before the plateau is reached. In other words, fresh motoneurones are 'recruited' into the sphere of action. The ascent of the myogram is due not only to fusion of successive contraction-waves within the individual fibres of the muscle ('wave-summation'), but also to the successive 'recruitment' of fresh motor units in the nerve-centres. The long gradual development of contraction-tension contrasts against the tension-rise at the opening of the flexor reflex (Fig. 10) or of any motor-nerve tetanus (Fig. 32).

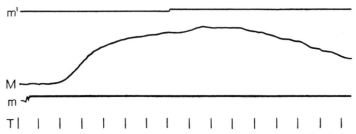

FIG. 31. 'Crossed Extensor' reflex elicited in vasto-crureus by stimulation of the contralateral sciatic nerve. M myogram; m onset of stimulus; m' end of stimulus. Time, 0·1 sec. Stim. freq. = 38 per sec.

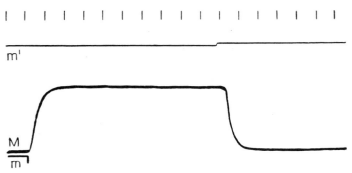

FIG. 32. Motor response from the knee-extensor by stimulation of its nerve. Time, 0·2 sec. Stim. freq. = 38 per sec. Lettering as in Fig. 31.

Further differences between this reflex and the flexor reflex are the greater smothering of stimulus-rhythm [116] and better maintenance of plateau level. Even when the rate of stimulation is quite low, fifteen or less a second, there may be little trace of rhythm in the myogram of the reflex, especially at the plateau (Fig. 33). Accompanying this smothering and related to it is found the presence in the electrical record of a number of small secondary waves between the large primary ones. The primary waves correspond to the rhythm of series of break-shocks which constitute the stimulus. The small or secondary waves denote asynchronous action currents in the muscle. Some of this asynchronism may be due to genuine asynchronous discharge of different groups of motoneurones. In other words, although the majority of motoneurones discharge almost together and produce the large primary waves in the electrogram, some motoneurones are out of step and discharge at varying intervals after the main group giving rise to smaller or secondary waves.

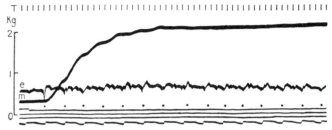

Fig. 33. Reflex response *m* of knee-extensor from stimulation of a contralateral nerve. Stim. freq. = 14 per sec. Time, 0·02 sec. The primary waves of the electrogram *e* are marked by dots.

But there is another cause for the asynchronism of the action currents. If any one motoneurone discharges more than once after a single stimulus, it will produce secondary waves in the electrical record as often as it discharges. This repetitive discharge is, of course, 'after-discharge'.[1] There is other evidence of considerable central after-discharge in the crossed extensor reflex [178], and so it must be concluded that the confused after-discharges of active motoneurones play a large part in the asynchronism of the electrogram. The secondary waves increase *pari passu* with recruitment and are more evident in the plateau than in the ascent [50, 97].

The propriety of dividing action-currents into 'primary' and 'secondary' waves when asynchronism is the cause of the difference may well be called into question. The present terminology is not adequate.

In flexor reflexes, secondary waves are probably entirely due to central after-discharge.[1]

iii. When recruitment is evoked by a stimulus of greater

[1] See footnote, p. 66.

frequency than twenty a second, the primary waves become less distinct because they are masked by secondary waves. This may happen also at the end of a long stimulation, even at a slow rate, for the secondary waves may be so well developed and frequent that the primary waves cannot be distinguished. When stimulation ceases, the reflex may continue undiminished sometimes for as long as a second before there begins a slow decline, indicating the gradual cessation of neurone-discharge. For what reason does the reflex thus continue undiminished for a time after the end of the stimulus? Two factors are concerned: (i) 'In the muscle with its afferent nerve intact a proprioceptive autogenous reflex adds itself to the reflex caused by the intrinsic afferents' [177]; (ii) 'There is also the "after-discharge" greater with stronger stimuli than weaker and referable directly to the externally stimulated extrinsic reflex arc.' This latter is not abrogated by deafferentation of the muscle. In part, therefore, the non-subsidence is due to there being a plateau of 'true', 'central', or 'repetitive' after-discharge. For example, a stimulus lasting five seconds elicited a response in a deafferented muscle with a plateau after-discharge lasting 0·2 second [97]. This after-discharge must be of central and not of peripheral origin. In part also the non-subsidence is due to the imperceptible blending into the plateau of a stretch reflex which 'takes over' from the crossed extensor reflex ('tonic appendage').[1] The stretch reflex disappears after deafferentation. If a preparation be used with marked decerebrate rigidity, i.e. with marked tonic after-discharge to the crossed extensor reflex, there will be little or no decline in the tension of the crossed reflex when the stimulus is intermitted for a short time. For instance in Fig. 34 the tension is maintained by the tonic appendage as well as by repetitive after-discharge. If the muscle is then deafferented, the tonic appendage is abolished and the fall in tension occurs earlier and more rapidly.

---

[1] These two features summed together can be called without prejudice 'after-action'. Although no precise definition exists of 'after-discharge' or 'after-action', it would seem better to restrict the term 'after-discharge' to true or central after-discharge, i.e. the repetitive after-discharge of nerve-centres after the first response of the centres to each stimulating shock. 'True' after-discharge is summed in this reflex with the 'tonic', 'postural' or 'myotatic' appendage.

This cutting of the afferent spinal roots of a muscle throws light on the function of muscular proprioceptors, as well as simplifying the problem of investigation. At the outset, the latent period is sometimes longer in the deafferented muscle. Two reasons are possible: (1) in acute preparations, trauma from the operation of deafferentation which appears as an inhibition; (2) prolongation of the summation period because there is no adjuvant stretch reflex. The latency once over, the

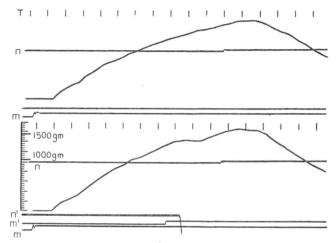

Fig. 34. Reflex response of knee-extensor from stimulation of a contra-lateral nerve. In the upper tracing the stimulation is continuous but in the lower tracing there is a lapse of 4–5 successive stimuli between *m'* and *n'*. *m*, onset of stimulus. *n*, end of stimulus. Stim. freq., 48 per sec. Time 0·1 sec.

contraction of the deafferented muscle develops with an abrupt rise different from the recruiting opening of the non-deafferented muscle, 'as though its momentum were less controlled than in the normal' [177], Fig. 35. In agreement with the myogram, the electrogram of the deafferented muscle is remarkable for the earlier appearance, greater frequency, and greater amplitude of secondary waves than in the non-deafferented muscle.

In some preparations, especially those in which there is only a small proportion of summed after-action due to the tonic element, there may be actual prolongation of after-discharge following deafferentation. Since the operation abolishes the tonic appendage, the prolongation can only be due to a lengthening of repetitive after-discharge ('central' after-discharge).

These features point to a release of the motor centres from some inhibitory influence. It seems probable that some of the characteristics of the extensor reflex are only accessory and can

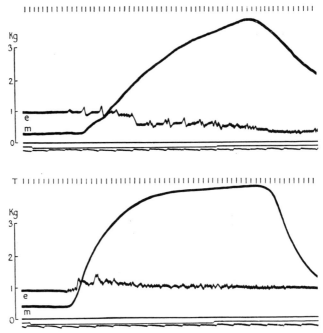

FIG. 35. Reflex response *m* of knee-extensor from stimulation of a contralateral nerve. Upper tracing, before severing dorsal roots. Lower tracing, two hours after cutting dorsal-root supply of muscle. Same conditions of stimulation throughout. Before deafferentation, the primary waves in the electrogram *e* are discrete. After deafferentation, secondary waves are evident, and primary waves are not. Time, 0·02 sec.

be stripped away by destruction of the proprioceptors. Thus the crossed extensor reflex, except in deafferented muscles, is inevitably blended with the stretch reflex since both are present in similar reflex conditions, e.g. in the thalamic or decerebrate or chronic spinal preparation. Since much of our knowledge of the crossed reflex is derived from non-deafferented muscles, proper allowance must be made for this complicating factor.

The bulbar centres in the customary decerebrate preparation also add to the complication. There is no reason to suppose that the extensor reflex and the stretch reflex each possess a private motoneurone pool. Motoneurones which take part in the stretch reflex probably also take part in the crossed reflex. Motoneurones recruited in the stretch reflex lie within the ambit of excitation of the crossed reflex, because during some seconds after the crossed reflex the stretch reflex is more easily elicited than before [122]. This effect declines gradually and subsides after 50 seconds. This greater readiness of the reflex centres to respond to impulses from stretch organs is due to increased central excitatory state which is residual after the crossed reflex. The two reflexes, therefore, engage closely related if not the same motoneurones. In result, the blending of effect is present during the elicitation of any crossed reflex in a non-deafferented muscle.

It is well known that when a motor nerve is stimulated, the muscle, separated from nerve-centres, develops an active tension which depends on the initial tension before contraction. But an extensor muscle in connexion with its nerve-centres appears to be especially responsive to high initial tension [117]. It is reasonable to suppose that the stretch reflex evoked by the high initial tension has already raised the central excitatory state of neighbouring motoneurones, but not to liminal value. Hence when the impulses arrive from the crossed side, liminal value is quickly reached. If a single crossed stimulus is found to be subliminal at low initial tension, it often becomes liminal at higher initial tension.

As has been pointed out, the coalescence of the crossed reflex with the stretch reflex is largely responsible for the long duration of after-action in the former, although it is clear from the reaction of deafferented muscle that part of the after-action is due to repetitive discharge of nerve-centres ('central' after-discharge).

This analysis of the blending of the reflexes is important for the light which it sheds on volitional movement. The stream of impulses descending the pyramidal tract may be regarded as analogous to the volleys in the afferent fibres of a crossed extensor reflex. A movement which is to be effective for an animal's need often should not cease abruptly but should change with smooth transition into posture. Posture is no less important than movement and, without smooth transition from one state to the other, ataxia will impose its disabilities on the muscular act.

As concerns functional facilitation from overlap of central connexions, the crossed extension reflex (after deafferentation) gives marked results [75]. Facilitation is frequent and often extreme between reflexes which must therefore be closely allied. Facilitation develops slowly and does not appear to reach its maximum until recruitment is almost complete. If one stimulus is withdrawn at that stage, its lapse is without result for 0·5 sec., as the plateau of after-discharge shows, and the effect lingers at the synapses, even for five seconds ('sustained facilitation' [75]).

'Rebound' [169].

'Rebound' may be described here conveniently, but it is not confined to extensor muscles or to this reflex. 'Rebound' is a reflex muscular contraction following withdrawal of stimulation of an afferent nerve-trunk. It often occurs if there has been inhibitory stimulation during the elicitation of a reflex, especially when the inhibitory stimulus is moderate in strength and duration. If the inhibitory stimulus is not strong enough or too strong or applied for a long time, 'rebound' does not appear and even under the most favourable conditions of experiment it is somewhat fickle.

The interval between the withdrawal of the stimulus and the appearance of the 'rebound' is much longer than the ordinary reflex latent period. It is often 0·2 sec. or more.

'Rebound' can also be effected by merely weakening as well as by withdrawing the inhibitory stimulus. Also it may be found that a weak stimulus which, when initially applied yielded inhibitory relaxation, yields 'rebound' contraction if it is immediately preceded by a strong stimulation. (See Fig. 59.) 'Rebound' is very easily inhibited by reapplying the inhibitory stimulus which evoked it or any other inhibitory stimulus (Fig. 36). 'Rebound' occurs in deafferented muscles and in flexor muscles also [34], but is demonstrated with especial ease in the extensor muscles of decerebrate preparations, when it often gives big contractions approaching maximum reflex tension. These may endure several seconds unless inhibited, and then decline slowly. The electrical record of 'rebound' resembles the plateau after-discharge of the crossed extensor reflex [97].

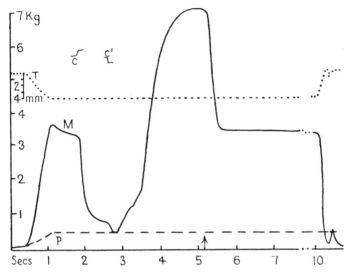

FIG. 36. Between *c* and *c'* the stretch-reflex of vasto-crureus is inhibited by faradization of the peroneo-popliteal nerve of the same side. Note the inhibition and the further fall, 'post-inhibitory' notch after *c'*. (The 'post-inhibitory notch' is followed by considerable rebound which, in turn, is inhibited at ↑ by gentle traction on Biceps femoris of the same side. See Fig. 21.)

'Rebound' is limited to observations with bared afferent nerve-trunk stimulation, and a nerve-trunk commonly contains afferent fibres of mixed central effect. 'If the reflex influence exerted by the stimulus during its application has been twofold, i.e. both excitatory and inhibitory, the "rebound" contractions might be due to the excitatory effect persisting longer than the inhibitory after withdrawal of the stimulus, just as with combined stimulation of the inhibitory and accelerator nerves to the heart the inhibition masks the accelerator influence during the stimulation but the accelerator influence comes clearly to light after cessation of the stimulus' [195]. See also p. 111.

2. REFLEXES OF IPSELATERAL EXTENSION

There are exceptions to the rule that in the decerebrate preparation stimulation of a hind limb causes flexion [42, 68, 163, 193].

i. The stretch reflex and the tendon reflex are demonstrably reflexes which can be excited within extensor muscles themselves. Light massage on the belly of an extensor muscle exhibiting decerebrate rigidity sets up reflex contraction within it. Kneading of the muscle can also sometimes cause reflex relaxation of it. Nocuous stimulation of a muscle, such as tearing or pinching, causes powerful inhibition of it. Mechanical or electrical stimulation of the proximal stump of the cut nerve of one head of the knee or ankle-extensor inhibits reflexly the other heads of the muscle [170, 171]. When the stimulus is weak, this inhibition is often preceded by a brief reflex contraction, especially if the tonic muscle be under stretch at the time. The slight contraction continues during the inhibition but is obscured by it. The contraction is the 'Residual Ipselateral Extension Reflex'.

In brief, the evidence from local manipulation of the extensor muscles themselves strongly confirms the view that there are two ipselateral reflexes obtainable from the muscles reacting upon themselves, i.e. proprioceptive, one excitatory, the other inhibitory.

ii. The extensor thrust in the spinal dog is elicited by stimulation of the planta [168]. Pressure is the only adequate stimulus, pressure on an area from which a nocuous stimulus would elicit only the flexion reflex [163]. The thrust is favoured by stretch of the extensor muscles, being facilitated by initial flexion of the limb. The thrust is a phase of the gallop in the spinal dog.

It is possible that two other reflexes excited from the same area, namely, the positive supporting reaction of Magnus, Blake Pritchard, and Schoen and the spring reaction of the thalamic animal [127, 128, 143, 153], are closely related to the same reflex mechanism.

iii. Mechanical stimulation of the skin over the upper two-thirds of the thighs and over the perineum can cause bilateral extension of the limbs. Flexion of the limbs favours its appearance. The extension reflex is much commingled with the nociceptive flexion reflex of the limb, rendering it uncertain of occurrence. In the chronic spinal dog, after previous extension of the limb, flexion results. These extensor reflexes are in part sexual reflexes.

iv. In preparations recently made decapitate, and periodically in other preparations where neck and labyrinthine reflexes are excluded, the crossed extension response is replaced by crossed flexion, and from one preparation to another varying mixtures of crossed inhibition of extensors and crossed extension may occur from one and the same stimulus. These variations are particularly noticeable in the fore-limb and are subject to numerous conditions, including the general state of the preparation, and can be produced by a large loss of blood and by other procedures.

DESCRIPTION AND ANALYSIS OF THE RESIDUAL IPSELATERAL EXTENSION REFLEX [65]. A. WHEN EVOKED BY TETANIC STIMULATION

Post-inhibitory notch in the crossed extensor reflex [97, 119, 121]. In the deep inhibitions of extensor muscles caused by stimulation of an ipselateral nerve there is often found a small residual excitation which often the strongest stimulation cannot inhibit. Records of muscle action-currents show that this excitation is a regular discharge following the rate of the inhibitory stimulus, and that with the cessation of this stimulus the discharge ceases rapidly, so that the muscle relaxes, sometimes completely, for an interval before recovery begins. Such residual excitatory ipselateral extension reflex in quadriceps is seen in Fig. 36. The final relaxation after the stimulus, the 'post-inhibitory notch', indicates that the excitatory ipselateral extensor reflex has a shorter after-effect than the inhibition which accompanies it.

Responses of slow and rapid muscles to ipselateral excitation when the background is a stretch reflex [65]. If the pale rapidly contracting ankle-extensor gastrocnemius and the red sluggish ankle-extensor soleus be examined in their relative reaction to this residual ipselateral extensor excitation, some facts relating to its distribution are revealed. With the two muscles both showing some stretch reflex, a very weak stimulus to a suitable ipselateral nerve causes a rise in tension in gastrocnemius and complete relaxation in soleus, Fig. 37. The increase in tension in gastrocnemius is sudden in onset and irregular in maintenance and shows a slight further increase when the stimulus ceases. Soleus shows a sudden fall, checked for a short time,

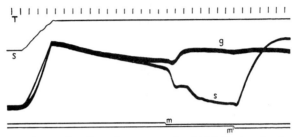

FIG. 37. A stretch reflex of gastrocnemius (thick line) and soleus (thin line). Repetitive stimulus to ipselateral peroneal nerve, secondary coil at distance of 14 cm. between *m* and *m'*. Time, 0·1 sec. *S*, fall of table.

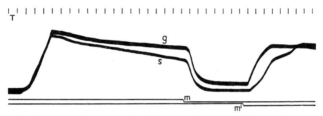

FIG. 38. Same experiment as in Fig. 37, coil 12, after improving state of inhibitory nerve by re-warming.

followed by progressive relaxation to a low tension. The check in the fall of soleus represents a small excitatory effect which is overwhelmed by the preponderance of inhibition, and is rarely seen well developed.

The excitatory effect is more often evident with weak stimulation or in preparations which show the excitation of gastrocnemius to a marked degree.

With a stronger stimulus, Fig. 38, both muscles relax rapidly to their inert tension, i.e. contraction ceases. Gastrocnemius, therefore, is more difficult to inhibit by an ipselateral stimulus than soleus and this obtains with all ipselateral nerves when the background against which the inhibition is pitted is the stretch reflex.

If there is no stretch in the muscle, the ipselateral nerves fail to excite, except the internal saphenous in the upper thigh, which produces an effect on soleus to be described later (pp. 77–8).

Responses of slow and rapid muscles to ipselateral excitation when the background is a crossed extensor reflex. If crossed extension be the background and there is no stretch reflex, it is difficult to demonstrate excitation by any ipselateral stimulus, for pure inhibitions are produced as a rule under these condi-

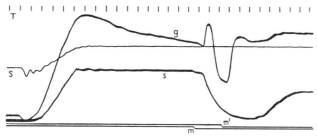

FIG. 39. Stretch reflex, gastrocnemius, upper myographic tracing *g*, soleus, lower tracing *s*. Stimulation to ipselateral peroneal nerve, between *m* and *m'*. *S*, indicator of table-fall. Time, 0·1 sec.

tions, but occasionally discharges may be seen in the electrical record, followed by post-inhibitory silence. But if there be a stretch reflex and crossed extension be added to it, the ipselateral stimulation produces residual excitation similar to that when stretch alone is the background. Passive stretch and the resulting stretch reflex appear therefore to be the facilitating factor and not mere active tension of unspecific origin. The difference is probably due to the fact that the crossed extension, in contradistinction to the stretch reflex, excites but little discharge in the motor units of gastrocnemius, and that not in the same motor units as ipselateral extension.

Response to excitation of different ipselateral nerves. The form which the residual excitatory reflex of gastrocnemius takes in any particular combination of background and ipselateral nerve varies greatly from one nerve to another and in the same nerve at different times. Often the excitatory reflex appears before the inhibition as a sharp peak followed by inhibition, Fig. 39, sometimes as a halt in the first fall of the inhibition, often as a faintly recruiting reflex early in the trough of inhibitory relaxation.

The rarely-seen excitation of soleus is evident under these conditions only as a halt in the inhibitory relaxation.

Difference depending on the background being a kinetic or static stretch. Some further points of difference between the reflexes

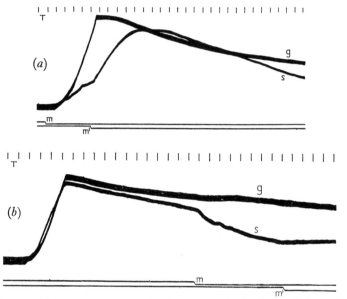

FIG. 40. (*a*) Same experiment as in Fig. 37, coil 16, stimulus applied early in stretch, and (*b*) late in stretch. Time, 0·1 sec.

are significant for their analysis. A stimulus to any ipselateral nerve which can evoke excitation of gastrocnemius and inhibition of soleus evokes a much more obvious excitation of gastrocnemius during the phase of increasing stretch (kinetic phase) than during the plateau (tonic phase). Soleus is inhibited in both phases, Fig. 40. Such differentiation is not obtained in the excitation of soleus by the internal saphenous nerve.

Rebound after the ipselateral reflex and its probable significance. A striking feature of the residual ipselateral reflex is the frequency with which it is followed by rebound. When a certain stimulus producing excitation in gastrocnemius and inhibition in soleus is increased in strength until gastrocnemius is also strongly inhibited, then on cessation of the stimulus gastrocnemius rebounds very sharply, but soleus remains completely inhibited, to recover only gradually, Fig. 41. The recovery in soleus is usually accompanied by further recovery in gastrocnemius. When the stimulus is further strengthened so as to abolish residual excitation in soleus, there is rebound in that muscle also, Fig. 39.

It can be surmised that suppression of ipselateral excitation by strengthening the stimulus causes rebound of short latency

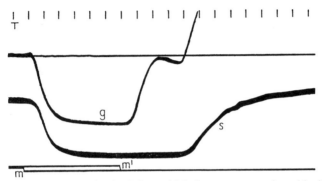

Fig. 41. Thalamic animal. Soleus, thick line, gastrocnemius, thin line. Stimulus to posterior tibial nerve between *m* and *m'*. Time, 0·1 sec.

and rapid development (Denny Brown). This type of rebound is so constant that the appearance of sharp forceful rebound following the stimulus may be taken as signifying that an excitatory effect has been produced but is kept inhibited by the stimulus. On the other hand, inhibition when uncomplicated by excitation, i.e. 'pure' inhibition, does not produce rebound. In fact it is probable that it is followed by gradual recovery, proportionate in delay of onset and in duration to the strength of the stimulus.

Differences between responses from stimulation of pedal and inguinal branches of the internal saphenous nerve. These differences are marked and are of considerable interest. The ipselateral internal saphenous nerve and often the obturator nerve, if stimulated very strongly in the upper thigh, even when the muscles are not stretched, causes a contraction of soleus but little or no contraction in gastrocnemius. The response in soleus usually recruits for a time so that a tension-plateau is reached which is not far short of the maximal contraction of the muscle, but in gastrocnemius the response reaches only a small tension and fatigues rapidly. The pedal and lower branches of the internal saphenous nerve fail to produce these reflexes.

If both muscles are stretched, they are deeply inhibited at first by stimulation of the proximal nerves with only faint evidence of excitation, but soon the recruiting excitation of soleus occurs with shorter latency than before and developing greater tension. This reflex of soleus is, therefore, also enhanced by stretch.

These differences show that there are two distinct types of ipselateral excitation in the hind limb, the one minimal in degree, widely distributed in areal source and affecting the pale, rapidly contracting gastrocnemius more than soleus, the other, just described, powerful and exciting the slowly-contracting red soleus and having an areal source restricted to proximal nerves. The reflex in pale muscles is almost entirely dependent on a previous stretch reflex and possibly for this reason is most evident in the decerebrate state. On the other hand, the reflex in red muscle is as evident in the spinal state as in the decerebrate and though enhanced by the stretch reflex, is independent of it.

Behaviour of Flexor Muscles. The flexor responses to ipselateral stimulation might well be expected to display the inhibitory counterpart of extensor reflexes. The only nerve possessing a relatively constant inhibitory effect on the flexors of the same limb is the posterior tibial nerve. Its effect occurs only on some of the units of any flexor muscle, Fig. 42, and then only when strongly stimulated. The effect is absent in some spinal preparations. This property of the posterior tibial nerve may be associated with the innervation on the pad of the foot and with the extensor thrust resulting from stimulation of that area. The effect is also produced but in much less degree from the higher branches of the same nerve, e.g. that to the posterior tibial muscles and in rare instances from the anterior tibial or peroneal nerve. The effect is never pure but is always mixed with strong excitation of other units, and the rebound which sometimes follows reveals repressed excitation of the same inhibited units.

Ipselateral contractions in the fore-limb [68]. The fore-limb reflexes are remarkable for the magnitude of their ipselateral extensor responses. The median and ulnar nerves are the most

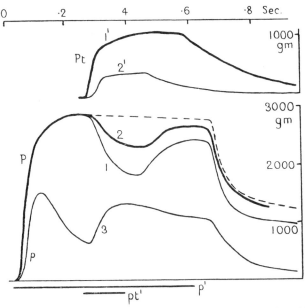

FIG. 42. Semitendinosus. Upper set of tracings: *Pt*, stimulation of ipselateral posterior tibial nerve alone; *1'*, coil distance 13·8 cm.; *2'* coil 15·5 cm. Lower set of tracings : *P*, stimulation of ipselateral peroneal nerve, during *p'*, coil 13·8 cm.; *pt'*, stimulation of ipselateral posterior tibial nerve, *1*, 13·8 cm., *2* and *3*, 15·5 cm.; *p*, peroneal, coil 22 cm. Broken line, control obs. without intercurrence of *pt'*.

powerful excitatory channels and their terminal branches excite the shoulder-extensor, M. supraspinatus. The contraction is of recruiting type. The contraction can be inhibited by stimulation of nerves more proximal, and even of the more proximal branches of the nerve provoking it, e.g. branches of the median nerve in the forearm. The ulnar and internal cutaneous nerves give responses exactly similar to the residual ipselateral responses in the hind limb with sharp powerful rebounds. Tetanic stimulation of the skin of those areas with stigmatic electrodes reproduces the same type. In the fore-limb the influence of the stretch reflex on ipselateral responses is very obvious and even the large responses produced from the median nerve require some slight initial stretch for their elicitation. Just as the distal ipselateral extensor reflex in the hind limb, so the fore-limb ipselateral extensor reflexes are not facilitated by the reflexes of crossed extension. In the fore-limb, too, all extensor reflexes are very much more evident in pale rapid muscles, such as the short head of triceps, while red slow muscles are inhibited by the same stimulus.

The differences in reaction between gastrocnemius and soleus, therefore, are not due to a possible flexor effect of gastrocnemius in flexing the knee, and the differences between these types of muscles are exemplified also by vastus lateralis and crureus, both pure knee-extensors.

We may infer that both in the fore and hind limb there is a type of extensor-exciting afferent which is concentrated in the distal part of the limb and in the distal branches of the nerves which supply that area and is less frequent in the branches near the base of the limb. But the hind limb shows additional extensor reflexes when stimulated near its base, because there adjoins and merges on to it the perineum, mamma, &c., with all their visceral and sexual significance.

DESCRIPTION AND ANALYSIS OF THE RESIDUAL IPSELATERAL
EXTENSION REFLEX. B. WHEN EVOKED BY SINGLE SHOCK STIMULI

If a single break-shock is applied to a suitable peripheral nerve, there occurs a small contraction with a few action currents, Fig. 43. This is the ipselateral extensor twitch. It is remarkable for the sharpness of its occurrence and disappearance in spite of a constantly long latency. The course of its event becomes apparent when two such break-shocks follow one another in the same nerve at varying intervals. The second break-shock, if it falls within the latent period after the first, delays all reflex excitation until, in turn, its own latent period has elapsed. There is in fact inhibition.

If the break-shock is introduced during any background discharge with a continuum of asynchronous action-currents, the
whole centre is inhibited and all discharge ceases, but begins
again after 45–65 σ.

The ipselateral extensor twitch occurs only in pale muscles.
When both red and pale muscles are examined together, with
the double string galvanometer, the pale muscle is found to

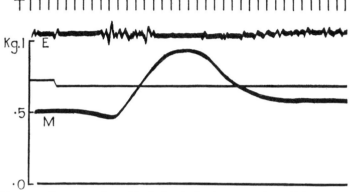

FIG. 43. Gastrocnemius. Single break-shock to posterior tibial nerve, at
fall of signal. *M*, myogram. *E*, electrical record. Time, 0·02 sec.

recover sharply after inhibition but the red recovers slowly and
gradually. The ipselateral extensor twitch is a rebound.

If then the ipselateral twitch from one break-shock is inhibited by a second break-shock as late as 60 σ after, what occurs
when the ipselateral stimulus is the series of break-shocks at
50 a second (20 σ apart) which provoked the ipselateral reflexes
discussed above? Such a series against a vigorous stretch background shows that at first there is complete silence in the string.
But towards the end of the interval preceding each stimulus
wave, small action-currents begin to break through and reach
full size slowly or rapidly according to whether the reflex
excitation is recruiting or *d'emblée* in type. In tetanic stimulation, therefore, the sequence of events is similar to the discharge
from a single stimulus except that summation of *c.e.s.* shortens
the latency of successive excitatory responses.

Each centripetal wave thus appears to add *c.e.s.* until neurone discharge occurs, although inhibition must sum all the time in much the same way. *C.e.s.* may accumulate up-stream in centres away from the locus of inhibition so that inhibition acts as a sort of barrage against the arrival of excitation at the motoneurone (Denny Brown).

Latent successive induction [66]. Just as a series of tendon-jerks is used to test inhibition and recovery from it (p. 93), so events may be tested in the reflex ipselateral extensor twitch. Using fore-limb reflexes, the tendon-jerk in supraspinatus is found to be inhibited if the tendon is tapped during the interval corresponding to the long latent period, but is full sized or even supernormal if it coincides with the appearance of the twitch. It is also inhibited if the tendon is tapped after the twitch, and afterwards makes the gradual recovery.

Again, if a nerve produces only a weak ipselateral excitation by a series of stimuli but no reflex response by a single break-shock, it leaves an effect which is concealed until sampled by a series of tendon-jerks. It is then found that a tendon tap at a particular interval of 45–60 σ after the break-shock elicits a very large but short-lasting jerk. This effect documents the process of rebound from an ipselateral volley as a subliminal process— 'latent successive induction'.

This has its counterpart in the hind limb. Gastrocnemius, for example, gives a much larger tendon-jerk by latent successive induction than in ordinary circumstances.

Herein lies an explanation of the curious differentiation which ipselateral extensor reflexes make between stretch and crossed extensor reflexes. Alone of all forms of stimulation, the residual ipselateral extensor reflexes facilitate and increase the tendon-jerks in pale rapid muscle, because without ipselateral excitation the tension receptors in pale muscle affect most of the motor units only subliminally so that they do not discharge. In other words, in pale muscle the stretch reflex which is just subliminal and the ipselateral extension which is also often subliminal from inhibitory barrage, facilitate one another when concurrent. But in pale rapid muscle crossed reflexes have a very high threshold, e.g. the crossed extensor response of gastrocnemius is poor and does not facilitate the jerk or stretch reflex. In slow red muscles, on the other hand, although there is overlapping of units in the stretch and crossed extension reflexes, stretch reflexes are paramount and the ipselateral stimulus facilitates very few units. This fundamental difference between the two types of muscle is emphasized by strychnine.

Action of strychnine. In a decerebrate animal in which the gastrocnemius and soleus muscles give the usual reactions (p. 73) to ipselateral stimuli against a background of stretch reflex, the administration of 0·08 mg. of strychnine per kg. of body-weight is followed in the course of the next few minutes by a gradual increase in the responses of gastrocnemius [65, 135]. Distal nerves, posterior tibial and musculo-cutaneous, first cause an increase in excitation and then, as the effect of strychnine advances, more proximal nerves do so. Soleus, however, continues to be inhibited by the same stimuli, and even if the dose is increased to the stage of convulsions, the inhibition is not reversed. At last the obturator and inguinal part of the internal saphenous nerves induce large ipselateral contractions in gastrocnemius which surpass the normal responses of soleus to inguinal stimuli. Soleus, meanwhile, still gives its recruiting responses to inguinal stimuli (p. 77), but its contraction is now dwarfed by contrast with the large response of gastrocnemius.

The 'reversal' effect of strychnine on the ipselateral extension reflex is therefore the excitatory enhancement of the distal ipselateral reflex which has its receptive focus in the apex of the limb. The responses of soleus remain un-'reversed' (Denny Brown).

Conclusion.

The afferents capable of exciting the ipselateral extension reflex are evidently wide spread. But in most stimulations of afferent nerves where the reflex rule of excitation of ipselateral flexors and inhibition of ipselateral extensors appears to hold, there are obscured contrary effects. It is the existence of these effects which enables any particular level of higher centres or any particular state of the co-ordinating mechanism to 'set' the lower centres in such a way as to constitute a 'neural balance' (Graham Brown).

VI

CENTRAL INHIBITION

Introduction.

WHEN the nerves of a limb are stimulated in any way, the flexor muscles of that limb contract reflexly—flexor reflex—while in the opposite limb the extensor muscles contract—crossed extensor reflex. The purposive character of such responses is evident; if an animal in walking pricks one hind foot on a sharp object, that foot is immediately withdrawn, i.e. flexed, while the opposite hind limb extends and supports the hind-quarters of the animal. Now if the nerves of the opposite limb are stimulated during the flexor reflex, the picture tends to be reversed. The simultaneous stimulation of both ipselateral and contralateral nerves might be expected to produce a contraction of all flexors and all extensors, so that the purposive character of the reflexes would be lost and an intermediate position maintained at the expense of a considerable amount of energy. Such needless antagonism between reflex responses might well be frequent under ordinary conditions of life, for many types of receptor organs from all and any of the limbs must continually be bombarding the reflex centres with impulses, some of which increase the *c.e.s.* in centres of muscles producing one movement, and others the *c.e.s.* in centres of antagonists. But such antagonism does not occur. The purposive character of simple reflexes, when they are simultaneous, is not lost but is maintained and co-ordinated as a functional whole. Superfluous and wasteful contractions are suppressed, *inhibited*, and harmonious action prevails (Principle of Reciprocal Innervation).[1]

The features of inhibition can be investigated by observing the

---

[1] So far as co-ordination is effected in the spinal cord, this Principle postulates that flexor centres are excited *pari passu* with the inhibition of extensor centres. For example, if the flexor centre is excited 100 per cent., the extensor centre is inhibited 100 per cent., i.e. is excited 0 per cent. If the flexor centre is excited 25 per cent., the extensor centre is inhibited 25 per cent., i.e. is excited 75 per cent., and so on. When, however, higher centres, especially the highest centres (cortical), are in control, the effect of the Principle may be much obscured.

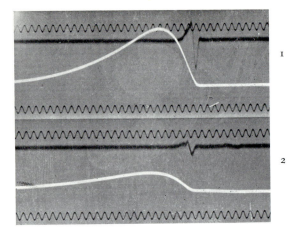

FIG. 44. *To be read from right to left.* Electrical and mechanical responses of Tibialis anticus muscle elicited as follows:

(1) Reflex elicited in response to a single break-shock applied to the ipselateral popliteal nerve.

(2) As in (1) except that a single break-shock was applied to the contralateral peroneal nerve 50 σ before the stimulation of the ipselateral nerve.

effect on a flexor reflex of a centripetal volley in a contralateral nerve. Since its field of action is in reflex centres, it can be demonstrated and measured only by its power of reducing or abolishing reflex discharge.

INHIBITION OF FLEXOR REFLEXES

Inhibition of a reflex flexor twitch by a single centripetal volley in a contralateral nerve.

A single centripetal volley in a contralateral nerve inhibits the flexor reflex evoked by a single centripetal volley in an ipselateral nerve; for example, if the volley of impulses in the inhibitory nerve (inhibitory volley) is set up 50 σ before the excitatory, the reflex response of the flexor muscle is diminished [26, 28, 83, 150] (Fig. 44). When the response is a reflex twitch, i.e. when there is no after-discharge, the inhibitory diminution must be due to prevention of reflex discharge of some moto-neurones. If a statistical average is assumed for the tension of an individual motor unit, the diminution in tension of the reflex twitch may be taken to be proportional to the diminution in the number of motor units activated, i.e. to the motoneurones inhibited. If the inhibitory volley is made smaller, fewer moto-neurones are inhibited. On the other hand, a larger inhibitory volley may inhibit all motoneurones, but only when the ex-citatory volley is small. With a weak reflex the number of moto-neurones inhibited by a given inhibitory volley is often larger than with a strong reflex. The motoneurones which respond in the weak reflex and then suffer inhibition are amongst those which, when taking part in the strong reflex, resist the inhibi-tion. In these motoneurones the prevention of reflex discharge by inhibition depends on the intensity of their excitation. If this is powerful, the inhibitory process may be present but without effect—a condition comparable with the subliminal central excitatory state. Moreover, the inhibitory process in any motoneurone is itself susceptible of grading, since an increase in the size of an inhibitory volley increases the inhibition of some motoneurones from a latent to an effective intensity. This condition is analogous to that existing in the excitatory process when a large excitatory volley produces reflex discharge of moto-

G

neurones which were in the subliminal fringe of a small excitatory volley.

Thus both the inhibitory and excitatory processes are capable of gradation in individual motoneurones, and the outcome depends on the relative intensities of the two processes. In some motoneurones the central excitatory state can be made so intense that even the largest inhibitory volley cannot prevent reflex discharge, while the converse is probably true, that in other moto-

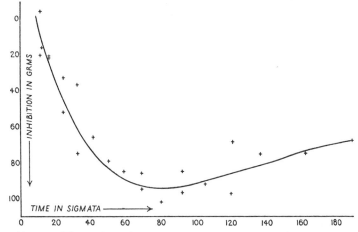

FIG. 45. The tensions of reflex twitches (ordinates) are plotted against the corresponding intervals by which the inhibitory volley precedes the excitatory (abscissae).

neurones the inhibitory process can be made so strong that the largest excitatory volley is ineffective. These results indicate that the modes of action of both processes are closely linked together.

With different intervals between the inhibitory and excitatory volleys the reflex twitch suffers varying amounts of inhibition [83, 150]. In Fig. 45 the intervals by which the inhibitory volley precedes the excitatory are plotted as abscissae, and the ordinates are the amounts in grammes of the corresponding inhibitions. When the inhibitory and excitatory volleys are set up simultaneously in the afferent fibres there is no inhibition, i.e. the inhibitory volley takes longer to produce its effect than does the excitatory. Even when the inhibitory volley precedes the excitatory by 6σ, evidence of inhibition is rare, its first appearance being usually at intervals of 6σ to 8σ.[1] When the interval is 30σ to 80σ, the inhibition exerts its maximum effect, and at longer intervals there is a progressive subsidence of the inhibition, but it is often still evident at 200σ. Since the ordinates can, at best, be considered as numbers of motor units inhibited, the intensity of the inhibition in any motoneurone bears no direct numerical relationship to the reduction of the reflex response. Nevertheless, it may be assumed that the larger the number of inhibited motor units, the more intense is the inhibition of the average motoneurone.

Thus the temporal course of inhibition of flexor reflexes is characterized by the comparative slowness of increase to a maximum and the still greater slowness of subsidence. These features are observed even when the inhibitory volley is so small that the degree of inhibition is comparatively slight. They do not depend on the choice of the ipselateral or contralateral nerves which are stimulated, and they are unaltered by deafferenting the muscle.

One reaches the conclusion, therefore, that the long duration of the inhibitory effect is strong evidence in favour of a central inhibitory state, c.i.s., which is antagonistic to the central excitatory state. It must not be forgotten, however, that the central pathway for contralateral inhibition probably includes at least one internuncial neurone. Histological study shows that fibres which enter the cord by the dorsal root of one side do not arborize around the cells of the opposite anterior horn [44]. It is generally agreed that inhibition is produced by nerve-impulses similar to those which give rise to excitation, and that inhibitory activity is manifested only at the region of termination of the nerve-fibres. Prolonged repetitive discharge of impulses in the internuncial neurone might give rise to a long lasting inhibitory effect even when the individual successive component inhibitions were quite brief. But this possibility is negatived by the experiments described in the next section.

Influence of excitatory impulses on inhibition [83].

If an excitatory volley is interpolated between an inhibitory volley and an excitatory volley, the response evoked by the

[1] The interval in the centres is not known accurately because the rate of conduction in inhibitory nerve-fibres has not yet been ascertained.

second excitatory volley is usually less inhibited than it is in the absence of the first excitatory volley. This happens even when the interval between the two excitatory volleys is too long for direct facilitation between them. The first excitatory volley, therefore, must enhance indirectly the response to the second excitatory volley by diminishing the inhibition. This is probably effected by inactivation of the inhibition of the motoneurones by the incident impulses of the first excitatory volley. Therefore some of the inhibition which is present at the time of incidence of the first excitatory volley must, in the absence of that volley, persist long enough to inhibit the response to the second excitatory volley. Such experiments show that inhibition persists for as long as 60 σ, and in many cases its duration is probably much longer. This persisting inhibitory condition may be called a central inhibitory state, c.i.s. The excitatory impulses responsible for the inactivation of the inhibition do not themselves give rise to excitation, for, if they did, a reflex discharge would be set up exactly as if no inhibition had been present. Thus it seems that c.e.s. and c.i.s. suffer a mutual inactivation.

At least three factors may be responsible for the time-curve of inhibition following a single inhibitory volley (Fig. 45):

i. Temporal dispersion of the incidence of the inhibitory impulses on the motoneurone. To this factor is doubtless due the increase of the intensity of the inhibition for a period as long as 60 σ after its onset.

ii. Persistence of the central inhibitory state produced by each inhibitory impulse. Owing to this factor there is a summation of the effects of successive inhibitory impulses.

iii. Subsidence of the inhibitory state. The eventual decline of the inhibition occurs when the rate of subsidence becomes greater than the rate of formation by the incidence of fresh inhibitory impulses.

Inhibition of a reflex flexor twitch by two centripetal volleys in a contralateral nerve [83].

When two similar inhibitory volleys in the same contralateral nerve are separated by an interval less than 60 σ, there is considerably greater inhibition of a reflex flexor twitch than from either

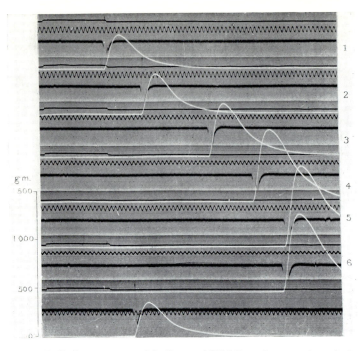

FIG. 46. Reflex responses of deafferented Tibialis anticus muscle evoked by an excitatory volley in the ipselateral popliteal nerve at various times during and after tetanic stimulation of an inhibitory nerve, the contralateral peroneal. The intervals before or after the cessation of the tetanic stimulation (shown by the signal line *above* the corresponding electrical record) were as follows: 1, 11 σ before end; 2, 78 σ after end; 3, 239 σ after end; 4, 345 σ after end; 5, reflex alone; 6, 424 σ after end; 7, 52 σ after end. The white lines of the myograph record commence *below* the dark lines of the corresponding electrical record. Time, 1 d.v. = 10 σ. Tension scale at side.

volley alone. As the distribution of effect of the second volley must be the same as the first, this added inhibition indicates that two inhibitory volleys inhibit some motoneurones which apparently are unaffected by a single volley. Latent inhibition, therefore, must be produced by either single volley, so that when both volleys are close together the summation of effect produces a degree of inhibition sufficient to prevent reflex discharge. In this property of summation the central inhibitory state resembles the central excitatory state.

When a volley in one contralateral nerve follows one in another nerve by a short interval, the total inhibition of the reflex flexor twitch is again found to be greater than when either is used alone. The maximum inhibition is usually produced when the two volleys are set up simultaneously. Then it may be greater in amount than the sum of the inhibitions produced by either contralateral volley alone. Hence these results also indicate that c.i.s. can be summed.

Effect of repetitive contralateral volleys [83, 196].

If the condition of the flexor centre be tested by an excitatory volley at various times during repetitive stimulation of a contralateral (inhibitory) nerve, it is found that the intensity of inhibition due to the latter increases progressively. The same method shows that there is a progressive diminution of the inhibition after the cessation of the contralateral stimulation (Fig. 46). The normal excitability of the flexor centre recovers after 0·5 second or more. The points of Fig. 47 show the amount of inhibition of the response to a constant excitatory volley set up at various times relative to a repetitive series of inhibitory volleys.

Effect of an antidromic volley on the central inhibitory state [83].

When an antidromic volley travels up the motor-nerve-fibres to motoneurones, there is a disappearance of c.e.s. from these motoneurones, and from this fact several conclusions have been drawn (p. 41). The long duration of inhibitory effect produced by a contralateral volley makes it possible to carry out similar experiments on the central inhibitory state.

If the antidromic volley is set up at various times between the excitatory and inhibitory volleys, the central inhibitory state is always unaffected by the antidromic volley. It might be thought that the antidromic volley would be prevented from reaching the seat of the central inhibitory state on account of the inhibition of the motoneurone itself. But it can be shown [202] that during such inhibition the axones of the motoneurones (motor-nerve-fibres) do not suffer any alteration in their excitability or conductivity, and that every motoneurone is subjected to the

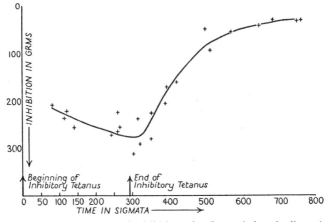

FIG. 47. The amounts of inhibition of reflex twitches (ordinates) are plotted against the corresponding time relations to a repetitive series of inhibitory volleys (abscissae). The beginning and end of the tetanic inhibition are shown by arrows.

influence of an antidromic impulse of normal intensity. Therefore it seems likely that the central inhibitory state cannot be modified by the antidromic volley. If it cannot, a most important and fundamental distinction between the central excitatory state and the central inhibitory state is established.

Inhibition of a reflex flexor twitch by a centripetal volley in an ipsilateral nerve [80].

Ipsilateral inhibition of the flexor reflex has been described on p. 35. Usually the inhibition reaches its maximum about 20 σ after stimulation of the ipsilateral nerve, and is still quite marked at 100 σ (Fig. 48). There is thus a very striking similarity of time relations between ipsilateral and contralateral flexor inhibitions. In both an antidromic volley passing up the motor-

nerve has no influence on the inhibitory process. When ipselateral inhibition is prominent, the response to tetanic stimulation of the afferent nerve is a single twitch followed by a sustained contraction of lower tension value, for the responses to
all afferent volleys after the first are reduced by the inhibition
from the preceding stimuli. This is the so-called 'jet' type of
reflex (Fig. 9). When inhibition is less pronounced, its presence

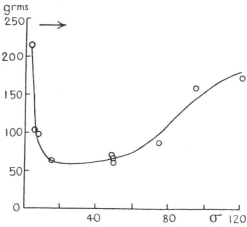

FIG. 48. The intervals between two stimuli (the 1st weaker than the 2nd)
applied to popliteal nerve (abscissae) are plotted against the corresponding
maximal tensions of the reflex responses (ordinates). The tension developed
by the reflex elicited by the second stimulus alone is indicated by the arrow.

is shown only by the tension of the tetanic reflex response
having an abnormally small ratio to that of the reflex response
to a single centripetal volley (p. 22); for some motoneurones discharge only once, and so do not develop their full tetanic tension.

*Inhibition of the reflex flexor responses evoked by repetitive
centripetal volleys.*

When a flexor reflex is elicited by tetanic stimulation, it is
never extensively inhibited by a single contralateral centripetal
volley, but a favourable background is obtained by having the
frequency of tetanic stimulus so slow that the stimulus rhythm
appears in the myograph record. Inhibition then shows itself
both in the mechanical and electrical responses, but its duration

is often so short that it cuts out only one of the primary waves of the electrical record together with the corresponding mechanical undulation. With higher frequencies the mechanical record fails to reveal inhibition although there may be a short period of relative quiescence in the electrical record. Such a short duration of inhibitory effect stands in marked contrast with the much longer periods found in testing for inhibition by a reflex twitch. The rapid repetition of the excitatory volleys evidently curtails the duration of the inhibitory process produced by the single inhibitory volley. The experimental observations from which Beritoff [18] concluded that the inhibitory process may have a duration of only 4 σ have been criticized from another point of view [83].

Inhibition of a tetanic flexor reflex by repetitive contralateral volleys is experimentally not a common feature in the spinal cat, but is more frequent in the decerebrate preparation. If contralateral volleys are set up during a flexor reflex, the usual result is an abrupt fall of tension to a fairly well maintained plateau. When the flexor reflex is not strong, all gradations of inhibition, from nothing up to totality, may be obtained by altering the strength of the contralateral volleys [175, 194], though frequently it is impossible to inhibit completely even a weak reflex. This grading is closely comparable with that obtained with single centripetal volleys.

When repetitive contralateral volleys are pitted against flexor reflexes of varying strengths, it is sometimes found that the weaker reflexes are completely inhibited while the very strong reflexes suffer no inhibition at all, and intermediate strengths are partly inhibited. In some preparations inhibitory volleys produce a considerable inhibition of a moderately strong reflex but are without any effect on a very weak reflex. In the latter case, the excitatory volleys can be only just strong enough to excite the motoneurones, and the absence of an inhibitory effect shows that hardly any inhibition can be incident upon them. But in the stronger reflex many of the additional motoneurones are inhibited. They must be subjected to a stronger inhibition than the former group. It is evident, therefore, that centripetal volleys in a contralateral nerve do not inhibit all motoneurones in the flexor centre to the same degree [59].

Inhibition of after-discharge.

A contralateral centripetal volley inhibits many fewer moto-neurones when applied during the stimulation-plateau of a tetanic flexion reflex than during the subsequent period of after-discharge, i.e. motoneurones are more easy to inhibit during the after-discharge than during the period of stimulation, because, in after-discharge, there is less 'central drive'. Thus a motoneurone presents a different resistance to inhibition under different circumstances [121] (see pp. 85, 100).

INHIBITION OF EXTENSOR REFLEXES

Since ipselateral centripetal volleys excite reflex discharges to flexor muscles and inhibit reflex discharges to extensor muscles

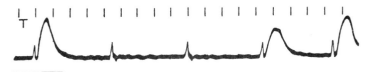

FIG. 49. Spinal preparation showing complete inhibition of the knee-jerk for a period of 0·8 sec. by a single break-shock applied to the ipselateral hamstring nerve at the point shown by the signal. Time, 0·1 sec.   *Note 28*

(Principle of Reciprocal Innervation), consideration will be given to their effect on the various types of reflex contractions of extensor muscles, namely the tendon reflex, postural contraction, and the crossed extensor reflex.

Inhibition of tendon reflexes.

In the spinal animal a single centripetal volley in a suitable afferent nerve, e.g. peroneal, abolishes the knee-jerk for some time (Fig. 49) [14, 155, 168]. The maximum length of time for this total inhibition of the knee-jerk is 2·0 sec. Usually a gradual recovery of the normal excitability begins 0·3 to 0·5 sec. after the inhibitory volley and is complete in 1 to 2 seconds. If the inhibitory volley is weak, inhibition is not complete and recovery is more rapid. The development of maximum extensor inhibition is practically instantaneous and the extensor centre recovers only slowly from inhibition (compare with flexor, p. 86).

Inhibition is complete even when the tendon tap is synchronous with the setting up of the inhibitory volley [95].

Inhibition of the decerebrate knee-jerk is a more involved reaction, since, in some circumstances, it is complicated by the effect of the centripetal volley on centres in the brain stem and by centrifugal volleys from these centres to the lower spinal centres. Larger volleys are needed to produce inhibition, and recovery is much more rapid, e.g. within 0·1 sec. [14].

Although the long duration of the inhibition of spinal knee-jerks strongly suggests that inhibition is a state capable of existing for a considerable time, i.e. a central inhibitory state, it is not a conclusive proof of such a condition. Since the spinal tendon-jerk can be obtained only when the muscle is under high initial tension [14, 95], it is possible that a considerable background of subliminal excitation in the extensor centre (from the tension receptors in the muscle) is necessary before it can be elicited. The prolonged depression of the spinal-jerk might be due to the slow building up of this background excitation after its removal by the inhibition. In the decerebrate preparation impulses descending from the brain stem effect a much more rapid building up of the background excitation and hence the shorter period of depression of the decerebrate knee-jerk. On the other hand, the increased susceptibility of these spinal centres to inhibition after spinal transaction may be due not to a lack of *c.e.s.* but to an increase of *c.i.s.*

Inhibition of postural contraction.

(*a*) *By a single inhibitory volley.* A single inhibitory volley produces a considerable relaxation of a postural contraction [156]. With different strengths of stimulus, the extent of the relaxation exhibits a grading as delicate as the flexor contraction which forms a part of the same reflex reaction [171]. The relaxation produced by a strong inhibition has a longer duration than that produced by a weak.

(*b*) *By two inhibitory volleys.* When a second volley, either in the same or in another ipsilateral afferent nerve, follows the first at a short interval, there is a further relaxation which is often much greater than that produced by the second volley alone. The mechanical record seems to indicate that many more motoneurones are inhibited. However, the electrical record often shows that there is for a short time an inhibition of *all* the motoneurones even when there is only a small relaxation in the myogram. Owing to the delay inherent in the relaxation of muscles after contraction (see p. 8), the reflex discharges reaching the muscle after the period of inhibition cause it to regain its previous contraction tension after a comparatively slight relaxation. The small relaxation conveys no hint of the

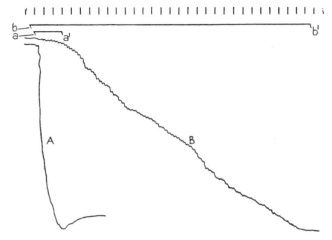

FIG. 50. Vasto-crureus muscle in a decerebrate animal. Inhibition of postural tone by break-shocks at 4 per sec. to the central end of the ipselateral musculocutaneous nerve. In *B* the stimuli were much weaker than in *A*. *a*, stim. on, *a'* stim. off, in *A*. *b*, *b'*, same for *B*. Time, 1 sec.

short-lasting total inhibition. A second inhibitory volley augments this small relaxation by prolonging the period of inhibition and so giving more time for relaxation. Also, it may inhibit motoneurones which apparently are not affected by a single volley.

(*c*) *By repetitive inhibitory volleys* [76, 171]. In Fig. 50 small repetitive volleys in an inhibitory nerve completely inhibit the postural contraction of muscle, but the time taken for this relaxation is longer than when the volleys are larger. The stepped relaxation in the former case is so very slow that its course represents approximately the progressive inhibition of the reflex centre, for the relaxation time of the muscle-fibres is relatively so short as to be inappreciable. With each volley more motoneurones are inhibited. The small extra amount of inhibitory effect in them sums with the previously latent inhibitory process to produce such intensity of inhibition that further reflex discharge is prevented. This progressive inhibition is called 'inhibitory recruitment' on account of its resemblance to excitatory recruitment. Thus inhibition of

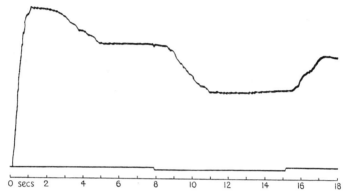

O secs 2   4   6   8   10   12   14   16   18

Fig. 51. Vasto-crureus muscle in a decerebrate animal. Inhibition of a stretch reflex by break-shocks at 50 per sec. to the small sciatic nerve during the time shown by the signal.

extensors is capable of summation in the same way as inhibition of flexors (p. 89).

If the repetitive volleys in the inhibitory nerve are made smaller still, the slow step-like fall may come to an end before the stretch reflex has suffered complete relaxation, and, although the inhibition is still in operation, a plateau of partial inhibition is reached after some seconds and maintained as long as the inhibitory volleys are continued (Fig. 51). It is probable that the same motoneurones are discharging throughout this plateau, and in them the inhibition remains latent though it is being added to continually by successive volleys. The reason is that excitation is also continually produced by impulses from the tension receptors of the muscle, and this excitation is sufficiently strong to overcome the inhibition. This state of affairs exists also during the inhibition of a crossed extensor reflex(see p.99), because this reflex is less susceptible to inhibition than muscle posture; for even the weakest inhibition, if repeated, commonly overcomes the mild excitation in posture.

If the sizes of two repetitive centripetal volleys in different inhibitory nerves are adjusted so that each alone produces a plateau of partial inhibition, they produce, when concurrent, a plateau of more complete or even total inhibition, and that sooner than with either alone. In any particular motoneurone there is a summation of the inhibitory effects of each afferent. In some motoneurones this is evidenced by inhibition when previously, from either nerve alone, there was none apparent. In other motoneurones there is a more rapid increase of inhibition so that reflex discharge is sooner prevented. Large repetitive centripetal volleys in an ipsilateral nerve immediately abolish all reflex postural discharge [63, 119], and the relaxation of the muscle then resembles the fall in tension after a motor-nerve tetanus.

Behaviour of the crossed extensor response to single excitatory and single inhibitory volleys.

When the quadriceps muscle of a chronic spinal animal is deprived of its afferent nerve-supply, the background excitation in the quadriceps centre is very much diminished, if not absent, since both proprioceptive impulses and impulses from higher centres have been cut off. In such a preparation, if experimental conditions are favourable, a single centripetal volley in a contralateral afferent nerve evokes a reflex contraction of the muscle. The reflex can be inhibited by a single centripetal volley in an ipsilateral nerve even if it precedes the contralateral stimulus by an interval as long as 150 σ. Since there is probably no background excitation in the extensor centre (see p. 151), this considerable duration of the inhibitory process is a true value. Even when the ipsilateral volley follows the contralateral by several sigmata, inhibition is complete. The latent period of the crossed extensor excitation must therefore be longer than that of the ipsilateral inhibition, as suggested by the observations on the short latent period of ipsilateral inhibition of the knee-jerk (p. 94).

Inhibition of the crossed extensor response to repetitive excitatory volleys.

(*a*) *By a single inhibitory volley* [121]. A moderately large single centripetal volley in an ipselateral nerve during the re-cruiting phase of a crossed extensor reflex does not produce a relaxation of the muscle, but only delays the rise of tension for a short period, about 0·02 sec. (Fig. 52). The increase of tension during recruitment is largely due to the continued addition of fresh motoneurones to those already discharging (p. 63), and in

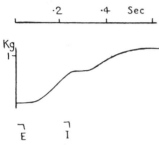

FIG. 52. Crossed extensor reflex in vasto-crureus muscle beginning at signal *E*. At signal *I* a single break-shock is applied to an ipselateral inhibitory afferent.

each of these motoneurones summation of the effects of the repeatedly arriving excitatory impulses eventually raises the *c.e.s.* to a threshold value. The short flat step in the recruitment curve probably shows that the moderately strong inhibition does not prevent the discharge of any of the motoneurones which were already discharging, but has for the moment stopped the recruitment of fresh moto-neurones. If the inhibition is stronger, a definite relaxation is produced, if weaker, the rate of recruitment is slowed.

If a considerable fall in tension is to be produced during the stimulation-plateau of a crossed extensor reflex, a fairly large inhibitory volley is necessary, and complete relaxation of the muscle may follow only a very large volley. For this event, all reflex discharge must be prevented until the muscle has had time to relax completely, i.e. for a period of about 200 σ, since reflex discharge during this time will hinder complete relaxation. It is remarkable that a single centripetal volley can have this prolonged action in the face of a continuous rapid bombardment of the reflex centre by excitatory impulses from the contralateral nerve. A moderately large inhibitory volley usually produces a very slight or no effect on the mechanical record of the reflex, while the electrical record often shows a short-lasting complete

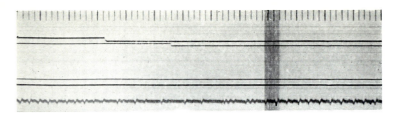

FIG. 53*a*. Electrical record of the responses of a single motor unit of an extensor evoked by stimulation of a contralateral nerve at a rate of 50 per sec. Between the two signals an ipselateral inhibitory nerve is stimulated at a rate of 65 per sec. Time, 0·02 sec.

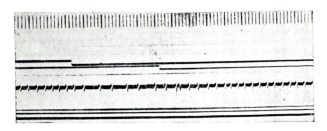

FIG. 53*b*. As in FIG. 53*a* in another experiment.

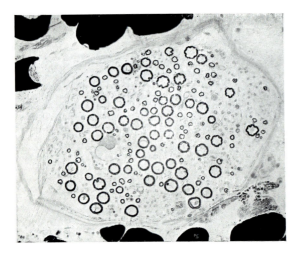

FIG. 67. Portion of nerve of M. biceps femoris, after removal by degeneration of all afferent fibres. Only ventral root (motor) fibres remain. Myelinate fibres $2\mu-18\mu$. $\times$ 320.

inhibition. After the inhibition the rapid bombardment of excitatory impulses restarts the reflex discharge before the muscle has had time to relax appreciably.

(b) *By two inhibitory volleys.* When a second volley, either in the same or another afferent nerve, follows the first at a short interval the inhibition is greatly increased. Even when either volley alone produces almost no relaxation the two volleys together often give a well-marked effect. Some of this increase is due in part to prolongation of the inhibited condition of the reflex centre, which allows a longer period for mechanical relaxation of the muscle (see p. 95). But summation of inhibitory effects probably operates as well, with the result that the two volleys together prevent reflex discharge of some motoneurones which were not inhibited by either alone.

(c) *By repetitive inhibitory volleys* [121]. A series of small inhibitory volleys gradually produces partial relaxation of a crossed extensor reflex, thereby showing that in the individual motoneurone there is a summation of the effects of each volley. Brücke [204] observes a phasic inhibition timed by interference of the excitatory and inhibitory rhythms. Larger inhibitory volleys produce quicker relaxation of the muscle, that is, the rate of inhibitory recruitment in the centres is increased. Very large inhibitory volleys cause an immediate cessation of discharge in all motoneurones, and the muscle relaxes as rapidly as at the end of a motor-nerve tetanus. That inhibition is able to quell instantly all reflex discharge shows that it must act on the reflex arc at least as far downstream as the point responsible for after-discharge. If it merely effected a block higher up, the result would be similar to a cessation of the excitatory volleys evoking the reflex, and relaxation would be delayed until the after-discharge had ceased.

In the crossed extensor reflex the rhythm of discharge of any particular motoneurone bears little relation to the rhythm of the excitatory volleys [10, 63], but depends on the rate of building up of c.e.s. in that motoneurone. Fig. 53 shows the electrical records of single motor units excited to respond at 20 per sec. by a series of contralateral volleys at 50 per sec. During a series of volleys at 65 per sec. in an ipselateral (inhibitory) nerve there is a reduction in the rate of reflex rhythm to about 7 per sec.

Rapid recovery to the original rate ensues after the inhibition [63]. Here, although the inhibition fails to suppress the reflex discharge, it nevertheless diminishes the rate at which the c.e.s. is built up, as is shown by the slower rate of discharge. On account of this slower rhythm the tetanic tension of the unit is considerably reduced, so that inhibition produces a fall in tension, although the reflex discharge still continues. Inhibition can thus reduce the tension of a reflex response by slowing the rate of firing of some units, as well as by suppressing all reflex discharge in other units.

Inhibition of after-discharge of crossed extensor reflex [121].

In the after-discharge of the crossed extensor reflex the bombardment with excitatory impulses is no longer intense, and, in

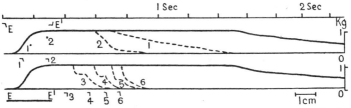

FIG. 54. Crossed extensor reflexes in vasto-crureus evoked by a stimulus applied between *E* and *E'*. In the upper figure a single break-shock is applied to an inhibitory nerve at either 1 or 2 (within the period of excitatory stimulation), and the effect on the after-discharges is shown by the corresponding broken lines. In the lower figure the inhibitory volley is set up at various points during the after-discharge.

consequence, the effect of inhibition bears a close resemblance to inhibition of the stretch reflex. Despite the identity of the motoneurones discharging in the stimulation-plateau and in the after-discharge-plateau complete inhibition of the latter is produced by a comparatively small inhibitory volley. Moreover, towards the end of the after-discharge-plateau, the later the inhibition the more marked are its effects (Fig. 54). According to circumstances, therefore, motoneurones vary in their susceptibility to inhibition.

After-discharge is affected in a characteristic manner by an inhibitory volley which is set up during the stimulation-plateau. Even though very little relaxation is produced at the time, the inhibition leaves its mark, for the after-discharge is curtailed (Fig. 54). This 'eclipse' of the after-discharge indicates that inhibition, while not producing a prolonged subliminal condition in excited motoneurones, at least is able to diminish the duration of their after-discharge. If a larger inhibitory volley is set up near the end of the stimulation-plateau, the resulting relaxation passes over to an after-discharge-plateau of reduced tension, i.e. those motoneurones which are most easily inhibited do not take part in the after-discharge. In some cases 'eclipse' is not

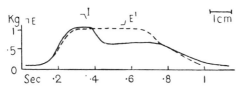

FIG. 55. Crossed extensor reflex in vasto-crureus evoked by a stimulus applied between *E* and *E'*. At *I* a single break-shock is applied to an inhibitory nerve. The broken line gives the course of the control (uninhibited) reflex.

evident, so that after-discharge is unaffected, and is identical in duration with the longest persisting after-discharge of the control reflex (Fig. 55). In these cases the motoneurones which exhibit the longest after-discharge are probably the least susceptible to inhibition.

General discussion on Inhibition [83].

As a summary of the experimental evidence on inhibition it may be said that:

(i) Centripetal volleys in ipselateral nerves as a rule excite reflex contraction of flexor muscles, and tend to inhibit reflex activity of extensor muscles. On the other hand, centripetal volleys in contralateral nerves excite reflex contraction of extensor muscles and tend to inhibit reflex activity of the flexor muscles.

(ii) The inhibitory process in motoneurones can be graded in intensity. It may be latent, i.e. subliminal [83, 188].

(iii) In a motoneurone summation of inhibition may be produced by successive volleys in one or more afferent nerves.

(iv) The inhibitory process is quantitatively antagonistic to the central excitatory state, *c.e.s.* In a motoneurone inhibition may slow the rate at which *c.e.s.* is being built up to threshold, i.e. it may slow the rate of reflex discharge, or it may prevent all discharge. According to circumstances, the same motoneurone varies in its susceptibility to inhibition. The more strongly it is excited the more difficult it is to inhibit.

(v) The antagonism between the central excitatory and inhibitory states is due to the mutual inactivation resulting from their interaction.

(vi) A single inhibitory volley sets up a central condition which can be detected for at least 100 σ. This duration is due partly to the temporal dispersion of the incident inhibitory impulses and partly to the duration of the central inhibitory state set up by any particular inhibitory impulse.

(vii) The central inhibitory state undergoes a progressive subsidence. This happens in the absence of incident excitatory impulses, i.e. without removal of *c.i.s.* by excitatory impulses.

(viii) The inhibitory process is unaffected by an antidromic volley 'backfired' up the motor-nerve-fibres.

(ix) Inhibition from any afferent nerve does not affect all the motoneurones of one muscle with a uniform intensity.

In the following respects *c.e.s.* and *c.i.s.* are analogous:

(i) They are only produced when nerve-impulses in the terminal branches of one neurone are incident on a neurone next Note 29 in series, i.e. at synapses. There is as yet no experimental evidence for the existence of inhibition with neurones other than motoneurones.

(ii) Both *c.e.s.* and *c.i.s.* undergo a gradual subsidence.

(iii) The *c.e.s.* or *c.i.s.* produced by one impulse sums respectively with the *c.e.s.* or *c.i.s.* produced by other impulses, from either the same or other nerve-fibres ending on that same motoneurone.

(iv) As a consequence of summation many grades of intensity of either *c.e.s.* or *c.i.s.* may be produced in a motoneurone.

(v) When *c.e.s.* and *c.i.s.* interact they suffer a mutual quantitative inactivation.

In the following respects *c.e.s.* and *c.i.s.* differ fundamentally:

(i) *c.e.s.*, if sufficiently intense, gives rise to the discharge of a nerve-impulse. No corresponding action is known for *c.i.s.*

It has no direct effect on the motoneurone—it merely inactivates   *Note* 30
c.e.s.

(ii) An impulse passing antidromically up a motor-nerve-fibre to a motoneurone inactivates the *c.e.s.* of that motoneurone, but does not affect the *c.i.s.*

The above differences between *c.e.s.* and *c.i.s.* have in all probability a common basis. Thus it may well be that *c.e.s.* acts as the sole intermediary between *c.i.s.* and the motoneurone, *c.i.s.* having no direct action [83].

No experimental evidence bears on the actual nature of *c.i.s.* It has been suggested that it is a chemical substance [14, 95, 150]. It may, however, receive its ultimate explanation in terms of physical chemistry, e.g. as the stabilizing of a surface membrane [190]. Certain it is that inhibition can exist independently of excitation.

VII

LOWER REFLEX CO-ORDINATION

By nervous co-ordination we may agree to understand that co-operation of nervous processes which secures with a normal muscular system the due performance of a muscular act. By due performance is here meant, since we are dealing with animal reflexes, execution of the act in such a manner as appears to an observer correctly to secure its end. Such normality will include normality of time relations, of spatial relations, and of tension development. Thus a movement must appear correct in speed, extent, direction, duration, and work done. Reflex acts of the simple kind considered in this book do not involve co-ordination of the highest and most delicate grades. For that reason they are likely to reveal explicitly some basal elements fundamental to all co-ordination. But to adduce due attainment of their end as an objective criterion for the co-ordination of reflex acts requires some preface here. Biologically the importance of a reflex is as an item of behaviour; hence biological study presents for each reflex the issue of its meaning as an animal act. On this rational basis the reflexes can be treated in a comprehensive functional scheme. It is, however, an aspect of their nature which has not been systematically regarded in this book; it can be found dealt with elsewhere [168]. Here the rough morphological scheme adopted separates them into uncrossed, crossed, spinal, decerebrate, &c., and has been followed as convenient. Such a scheme is less inappropriate for function than might at first seem, largely because reflex difference between flexors and extensors [160] does document itself in such a scheme, and is persistently significant. Within its arrangement we take such functional meanings as are obvious, to use them as criteria of effective reflex performance, and thus of reflex co-ordination.

We have to be circumspect. The laboratory usage for obtaining reflexes is often direct stimulation of bared afferent nerves, a plan which eschews selective excitation of specific receptors and precise knowledge of the receptive field, and thus renounces serviceable guides to the functional purpose of the reflex.

Further, an isolated muscle under myograph and galvanometer often yields, examined by itself alone, little evidence, and that equivocal, as to the meaning and general co-ordination of the full reflex act for which the muscle is part agent. Again, the collection of afferent fibres in a nerve-trunk, especially in one of considerable size, is drawn from receptors of such various species and place, superficial and deep, that its direct stimulation, especially if strong, cannot represent with purity the provenance of any normal natural stimulus. Direct stimulation of bared afferent nerve does, however, present certain advantages in reducing complexity arising from receptor organs. Also, the electrical stimulus, although even in its application to actual receptors generic rather than specific, does provide the experimenter with nicety of adjustment in strength and time. An objection attaching to the electrical stimulus for evoking reflexes lies in the circumstance that the relative heights of threshold of the various afferent nerve-fibres to that stimulus must depart widely from the distribution of threshold heights among the receptors to which those afferent fibres correspond, and therefore from the relative excitability of those fibres themselves under natural stimulation.

Some measure of caution is necessary, and brief mention will now be made of certain types of reflex result, derivable from direct electrical stimulation of bared afferent nerve, which are likely to be false guides if accepted as instances of normal reflex co-ordination.

I. CONCEALED REFLEXES

Each afferent nerve presents a dominant reflex. This reaction when the nerve is stimulated directly may obscure others concomitantly excited [94, 193, 195]. If the nerve be large and the stimulus strong the net reflex result on a muscle or group of muscles will be an admixture and may be self-contradictory and in so far too suspect to be taken as a pattern of normal co-ordination. The 'jet' form of the spinal flexion reflex can serve as an example (Fig. 9). This is excited from large afferents, e.g. from the foot or hamstring muscles; its rapid and powerful opening contraction is not maintained but early dwindles to a trifling remainder; this then continues as long as the stimulus lasts.

The afferent fibres stimulated include along with those that excite the flexor muscle others which excite the extensors and inhibit the flexor. These latter cut down the excitatory effect of the former: in other words an extensor reflex lies concealed under the flexor reflex.

Concealed inhibition obtaining in one afferent nerve can often be detected by concurrent stimulation of another. The con-

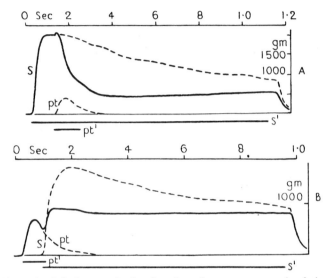

FIG. 56. Spinal *tensor fasciae femoris*; reflex response to stimulation of *internal saphenous* (*s'*) with in *A* an intercurrent stimulation of *popliteal* (*pt'*), in *B* a partly preceding stimulation of popliteal. The popliteal evokes a mixed but predominantly inhibitory effect which latter is revealed by a diminution in the contraction responses to internal saphenous nerve. In both, broken line above, control reflex from *s'* alone. Broken line below, reflex from *pt'* alone.

traction excited by the latter is then found to be diminished during the stimulation of the former. Thus, with the spinal muscle *tensor fasciae femoris*, the popliteal nerve gives reflex contraction of the 'jet' type. By combining this with stimulation of the internal saphenous nerve the reflex action of popliteal in the flexor is shown to be in fact mainly inhibitory [52]. Its reflex contraction in the hip flexor, *tensor fasciae*, conceals a reflex inhibition of the same muscle pertaining to an extensor reflex. That these reflexes although coincident are mutually destructive argues against accepting such gross admixture of them as instances of normal co-ordination.

Again, with such admixture stronger stimulation of one and the same bared afferent may yield in a sample muscle less contraction than did weaker stimulation, or may replace contraction by immediate and considerable relaxation. This latter is an example of what is called 'reversal' [193].

(i) *Reversal of reflex effect.*

'Reversal' is germane to concealed reflexes. It is met with in several forms: (a) reversal under change of strength of stimulation of the same afferent nerve [193, 194]; (β) reversal under continued and unaltered application of the stimulus [193]; (γ) reversal after exhibition of a drug, e.g. chloroform [192], strychnine [135], the stimulus and nerve remaining the same; (δ) reversal conditioned by altered initial state, e.g. posture of the limb [172, 161], the exciting stimulus and its locus remaining unaltered.

Progressive increase of the stimulation of a given afferent nerve and the resulting increase of contraction-response of a test muscle which it activates show, in some cases, a relation too bizarre to be accepted as exemplifying normal co-ordination [193]. Thus, the effect of a graded series of stimulations of internal saphenous or of peroneal as afferents can be as follows on the ipselateral tonic vasto-crureus: at threshold, contraction; with less weak stimuli, more marked and steeper contraction changing under unaltered continuance of the stimulus into gradual relaxation. With further increase of stimulus an initial contraction passing quickly into rapid inhibitory relaxation. On still further increase of stimulus no initial or other contraction but a swift and profound inhibitory relaxation.

In Fig. 57, faradization of the peroneal afferent excites tonic contraction in both right and left knee-extensors [179], but strengthening the stimulation, while it causes increased contraction of the crossed extensor, replaces that of the ipselateral by prompt and considerable relaxation. Here in the ipselateral reflex the response to the stronger stimulus conceals that belonging to the weaker. The weak reflex cannot bear the same functional meaning as the stronger being tonic and bilaterally symmetrical instead of phasic and asymmetrical; it is contributory to standing [179], which the asymmetrical response cannot be. The 'standing' is the weaker reflex and becomes masked. The stronger stimulation of the bared afferent therefore evoked a complex of two functional reactions, partly incompatible, artificially compounded in the same muscle [193]. The result is not utterly '*in*co-ordinate'. Excitatory summation and inhibitory summation and central interaction between them have

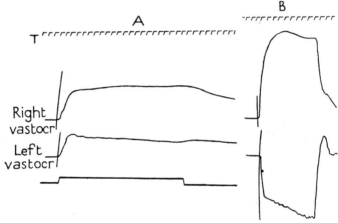

FIG. 57. Decerebrate vasto-crurei right and left. In *A*, weak stimulation of the left peroneal afferent; in *B* stronger but still moderate stimulation of the same afferent. Time, 0·2 sec.

contributed to it, and they can be mutually co-ordinative. But here the result is faulty in the sense of misexecuting one act by reason of simultaneous confusion of it with another. The co-ordinating mechanism is supplied with wrong ingredients; the same instrument is driven to play two different tunes at once. The disorder is faulty correlation [105] rather than inco-ordination.

Such cases of 'reversal' are not rare. One and the same afferent nerve can contain two sets of fibres which produce opposite reflex effects on the musculature. Thus the plantar nerves contain, besides fibres from nociceptors of the foot which inhibit the limb-extensors, fibres from receptors for harmless pressure on the planta which excite the extensors [163]. Again, the extensor muscle contains proprioceptive organs which on their mechanical stimulation by their own muscle excite reflex contraction of it (autogenous excitation) [166, 170], and the same muscle contains also other proprioceptive organs which on being mechanically stimulated by their own muscle reflexly inhibit it (autogenous inhibition) [170, 173]. The afferent nerve-fibres from both these antagonistic sets of proprioceptors within the muscle are gathered up together in the nerve of the muscle along with the motor-nerve-fibres, making one nerve in common. With an admixture of that kind subjected to graded electrical stimulation, one set of the reflexly opposed afferent fibres may predominate among the larger (i.e. low threshold) fibres of the afferent nerve and the other set among the smaller (i.e. higher threshold). In the instance above, excitatory fibres predominating in the large fibre group could explain why a threshold stimulus gives contraction, with little or no inhibition; and, if inhibitory fibres predominate in the medium and small calibre group, inhibition will predominate under such increased stimulation as includes these latter. That the result even under full stimulation may still show some initial contraction is intelligible because the large calibre fibres being quicker conductors will *ceteris paribus* provoke their central result earlier; often, however, the initial contraction entirely disappears. Further, one form of stimulus may suit one kind of nerve-fibre better than another.

It is, however, not intended to suggest that *every* case of 'reversal' of reflex effect under continuance of the same stimulus is *per se* an artefact or evidences inco-ordination. A reflex reversal given by a natural stimulus and offering no ground for rejection as inco-ordinate is furnished by the usual demonstration of the 'lengthening reaction' [173, 177]. There the knee-extensor is in decerebrate rigidity: passive flexion of the knee then initially encounters resistance, partly due to the excitatory autogenous reflex of the muscle itself already in action and partly due to enhancement of that by the additional stretch bringing in further proprioceptors excitatory of the muscle. Then under further persistence of the passive flexion inhibitory relaxation, autogenous inhibition, supervenes. Those proprioceptives of the muscle which are inhibitory of the contraction of the muscle itself, i.e. of their own muscle, are thus brought into play by the further stimulus. An inhibitory proprioceptive reflex supervenes upon an excitatory one. This supervening inhibitory reflex has its excitatory concomitant in the crossed fellow limb where contractions of the paired fellow muscle vasto-crureus (Philippson) [137] and of soleus are evoked.

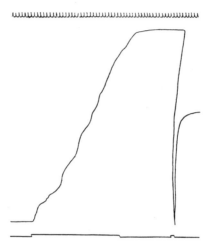

FIG. 58. Decerebrate vasto-crureus. Two reflex responses to stimulation of the same afferent nerve (ipselateral popliteal). The earlier and longer stimulation was by weak galvanic currents from a rheonome alternating in direction at 22 per second; this gave 'tonic' contraction. The later stimulation was a break-shock series from an induction coil at 30 per sec. through the same electrodes (non-polarizable) for somewhat less than one second; this gave immediate inhibitory relaxation. Time, 1 sec.

Again, the proprioceptive reflex excited by active contraction, a 'natural' stimulus, of the hamstring muscles provokes in vasto-crureus a mixed reflex, concealed excitation accompanying dominant inhibitory relaxation (Cooper and Creed) [55]. Again, the clip stimulus, a 'natural' stimulus, applied to a hind-foot digit of the spinal dog, excites protective flexion; but that flexion, under unaltered continuance of the stimulus, is quickly followed by rapid irregular alternation of extension-adduction and flexion-abduction, which may free the foot. Again, the reflex stepping of the fellow hind limb which accompanies the nociceptive clip reflex is itself a rhythmic reversal reflex. Clearly

not every reflex reversal under a continued stimulus is artificial
or inco-ordinate.

Nevertheless electrical stimulation of a bared afferent nerve
commonly has for its reflex result a clash of interaction between
receptors naturally opposed, a clash which natural stimuli do
not occasion. In this clash one of the opposed components
tends to conceal the others. Each considerable afferent nerve
presents a dominant reflex which may mask its competitors
[191, 193]. That dominance is itself a compromise between
conflicting reflexes. In an above instance the concealed ipselateral extension reflex was only partly submerged. There are
instances less facile to detect—especially where the concealed
reflex is inhibitory. Terminal rebound following on reflex
contraction is commonly accepted as a sign of a 'concealed
inhibitory reflex', so often does an outburst of reflex contraction
follow the production of strong inhibition.

(ii) *Rebound.*

The reflex effect of an afferent nerve, stimulated as such
directly, may, on withdrawal of the stimulus, be followed not
by mere lapse of the reaction but by outbreak of fresh activity.
This last may be opposite in sense to what had preceded, or may
be an enhancement in the same sense. This terminal phenomenon in its various forms is called 'rebound' [169]. Points
regarding it are [169, 34]: (1) it occurs both in the spinal and in
the decerebrate preparation; (2) deafferentation of the muscle
does not preclude it; (3) the stimulation must be well above
threshold; (4) it may ensue even on a single-shock stimulus—
commonly with a tetanic stimulus there is a favourable duration
of the stimulus for evoking rebound, and shortening this much,
or lengthening it much, excludes the rebound; (5) actual change
either in length or tension of the muscle is not essential or
important as a precursor for the 'rebound'; (6) the latent
interval exhibited is always long, often much longer than
ordinary reflex latencies; (7) the duration of the rebound itself
is variable but never very brief; its onset is quicker than its
subsidence; (8) it can be obtained by merely reducing in
strength, instead of withdrawing, the stimulus, and the strength
of stimulus which then allows the rebound is that which

initially produced the opposite effect to the rebound [172]; (9) it is easily inhibited [181], like after-discharge. Electrically, its muscle-response resembles that of after-discharge [92, 97].

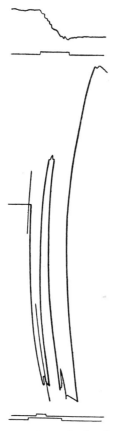

FIG. 59. Decerebrate vasto-crureus. Top figure: weak break-shock series applied to afferent ipselateral peroneal, and causing weak inhibitory relaxation of the tonic muscle. Lower figure: the stimulation strengthened by short-circuiting a resistance in the primary circuit but otherwise similar and delivered through the same unshifted electrodes; this causes stronger inhibitory relaxation. Then the stimulus is reduced to the strength it had in the top figure; it now produces contraction instead of relaxation. Finally the stronger stimulus is reverted to and gives inhibitory relaxation, followed on complete withdrawal of the stimulus by terminal rebound.

Types of terminal rebound are: (1) outburst of contraction following cessation of an inhibitory relaxation; (2) increase of contraction following a moderate contraction; (3) increase of relaxation (inhibitory) following a moderate inhibitory relaxation. The view has been put forward that, like reversal, 'rebound' is to be accounted for by admixture of afferent fibres [94, 193, 195, 205], excitatory and inhibitory respectively, and of different threshold in the same stimulated nerve-trunk. Points (2), (3), (6), and (8) especially support that explanation and none of the facts are incompatible with it. The explanation supposes central opposed effects dissimilar in time relations, the one appearing earlier, the other persisting the longer, with an intervening period of common action during which compromise obtains. The persistence of the inhibition, e.g. Fig. 56, harmonizes with the long duration of inhibition in general; spinal examples of such rebound are not infrequent. The persistence of excitation subsequent to inhibition, giving the rebound so usual in decerebrate preparations especially along with decerebrate rigidity, argues a remoter or prespinal seat for such persistent excitation.

Rebound is, however, not restricted to artificial stimulation or to stimulation of mixed afferent nerves. It can be a sequel to 'natural' stimulation. The jaw-opening [22, 183] reflex (decerebrate cat) is executed by contraction of digastricus accompanied by reciprocal inhibition of the powerful temporalis and masseter. Elicitable by broad pressure on the upper teeth and palate, it is followed immediately on removal of that stimulus by vigorous closing of the jaw from 'rebound' of the previously inhibited jaw-closers. With a series of stimuli, therefore, a 'biting' action results; the openings occur with the stimulations, the closings by strong rebounds between the stimulations. Reclosure when there is something between the jaws to bite upon brings into reoperation the jaw-opening stimulus. A rhythmic biting reflex thus maintains itself until the pabulum is gone.

The point here, however, is that rebound, with its seesaw of effect and its conflicting inhibition and excitation, is, when ensuing on stimulation of a large naked afferent nerve, like 'reversal' itself, traceable to 'concealed' reflexes and to the concurrent stimulation of opposed afferent fibres in a manner too gross to be acceptable as a normal co-ordination. The laboratory plan of obtaining reflexes by direct stimulation of bared afferent nerve is for some analyses excellent; but it is unnatural and certain reflex artificialities derive from it. Its results have therefore to be used circumspectly; though for the prosecution of reflex analysis in general it has furnished data of inalienable value. Its results, even when questionable as examples of normality, may yet instructively illustrate elemental processes of co-ordination at work on an abnormal basis.

II. QUANTITATIVE ADJUSTMENT OF REFLEX CONTRACTION

Among requirements which co-ordination must satisfy one, which seems as fundamental as any, is adjustment of what may be termed quantity of contraction. On this rests adjustment of extent and speed of movement, and of work or mechanical resistance commensurate to demand. Since every reflex act employs not one only but a number of muscles the quantity of contraction it adjusts is plurimuscular in distribution. A step towards analysis of this adjustment of quantity is to determine its component in the individual muscle. The myograph and galvanometer can do this. They show that a reflex deals with the muscle as a collection of additive units, the motor units defined earlier (p. 6). On this basis a reflex grades its activation of the muscle in two ways: (a) by operating fewer or more of the units; (b) by intensifying or lessening the degree of tetanic contraction of the individual unit.

Reflex scale of adjustment.

A reflex fractionates its muscle. This fractionation is based on the spinal motoneurone. Its limit of fineness in the muscle is set not at the individual muscle-fibre but at the individual motor unit, each such unit comprising many muscle-fibres, e.g. some 150 muscle-fibres [48] in (p. 16) cat. An advantage of the 'motor unit' over the individual muscle-fibre as unit of functional contraction is the mechanical one that the muscle-fibres of the unit form a lengthwise group which even in long muscles pulls on tendon directly and escapes the yielding intervention of slack muscle [49]. As to the least number of motor units employed it seems certainly to descend to 2 or 3 [78]; thus a single-shock stimulus of low value will evoke a 10 g. reflex twitch (*tib. ant.*) in a muscle comprising some 330 motor units, and giving a maximal motor twitch developing some 1,000 g. The upper limit of the number of units activated in the given muscle varies with the particular afferent nerve employed. It would be helpful could we assess the relative number of motor units engaged in variously graded reflexes; to do so presents difficulty. Advantages a twitch reflex would offer for the purpose are offset by the circumstance that such contraction when confined to a few units and submerged in an elsewhere inactive muscle is at serious disadvantage for approximate isometry of record. Moreover a single afferent stimulus, e.g. a single centripetal volley, fails to activate the full number of motor units which the same afferent nerve can activate under tetanic repetition of the same stimulus. Of reflexes the spinal flexion reflex offers the best chance for an estimate. With this reflex the tetanic rate employed for stimulation of the afferent nerve commonly secures a fairly corresponding rate of centrifugal discharge. Full tetanic contraction of those motor units which are reflexly excited is thus obtainable by a repetitive stimulus of sufficient rate. Indeed by full tetanic stimulation of a large afferent the reflex tetanus may occasionally develop the full maximal tetanic tension of the muscle [51, 52, 71], thus furnishing proof of complete tetanic contraction of every motor unit in it. With the flexion reflex an estimate has in fact been attempted of what fraction of certain flexor muscles of the limb is at the reflex disposal of this or that afferent nerve of its own limb. Approach is thus made toward what proportion of the motoneurones of the muscle is available for each of the afferent nerves excitatory of it. In deriving this proportion we remember that even under maximal stimulation of the afferent nerve some of the motor units engaged will, in the majority of instances and especially where the afferent is of small effect, not be driven to their full tetanus. The ratio of reflex contraction to maximal contraction will therefore understate the actual proportion of engaged motoneurones. Where the average tetanic contraction-value of the individual motor unit is known, the number of motor units at the disposal of the afferent nerve can be approximately assessed (p. 23). In the aggregate of motor units composing a muscle the fractions belonging to various individual afferent nerves overlap largely. The motoneurones operated by a large afferent may include the whole of those operated by another afferent nerve anatomically distinct from it.

The sum of the largest reflex contractions severally obtainable from the branches of an afferent nerve greatly exceeds the largest reflex contraction obtainable from the parent nerve composed of those branches. The increments of reflex contraction which accompany successive additions of fibres stimulated in a given afferent nerve will *ceteris paribus* decrease if for no other reason than that the fresh fibres added are as to their central terminations overlapped more and more by afferent fibres already in action. The same relation obtains when a skin area used for reflex excitation is successively enlarged; to double the skin area does not *ceteris paribus* double the reflex response.

Each increase of the stimulus of the afferent nerve, bringing enlargement of the centripetal volley, widens the fractional field of excitation in the motoneurone pool of the muscle. But the enlargement proceeds by increase in density of central excitation as well as by widening of the area excited. Central convergence and consequent summation make themselves felt throughout. Even at threshold and among afferent fibres belonging to two separate though adjacent nerves it is central interaction which establishes the actual threshold itself [190, 77]. The reflex threshold is therefore a *central* threshold, i.e. not the threshold of the peripheral afferent nerve. Such central interaction occurs between separate nerve-trunks and in the very genesis of their conjoint fractional field of excitation. Even more does it accompany the growth of the fractional field under increase of stimulation of a single nerve or during extension of a stimulated and continuous receptive field. To augment a reflex by increasing the stimulation of an afferent nerve already under stimulation and to augment it by concurrent stimulation of another afferent nerve are therefore two not very different steps. In either case, even where the change in afferent stimulation is purely one of extensity, i.e. number of fibres, the concomitant central change will, because of central overlap of the excited terminals with consequent summation and its effects, be a change of intensity as well as of extensity in the motoneurone pool of the muscle. To increase or reduce the number of motor units activated always involves changes in the intensity of excitation of motor units other than those actually recruited or shed. In the case of 'natural' stimuli a change of extensity of the stimulus is commonly accompanied by change of intensity; then the centripetal stream of impulses becomes not only wider but more frequent, i.e. the individual trains of impulses come to consist of impulses following more closely one on another. Reflex adjustment by extensity, i.e. number of motoneurones engaged, and by intensity, i.e. grade of excitation of the individual motoneurone, are thus more than ever associated.

Mention of the reflex centre as a summation apparatus hardly needs amplification here. Summation, the process, and evidence of it as a 'central' event, have been traced earlier (p. 31). There is summation of excitation at the motoneurone. The rate of firing of a motoneurone, often disparate from that of the centripetal volleys launched upon it, yet depends on the quantity of impulses arriving in a given time. Their excitatory effect is summed; the rate of discharge of the motoneurone rises with increase of the centripetal impulse-stream. That increase can be due to increase (a) in the number of active channels converging upon the motoneurone, or (b) in the number of impulses conducted in unit time per individual afferent channel. The 'principle of convergence' takes effect mainly through the former; intensity of adequate stimulus mainly through the latter.

Grades of reflex excitation.

The motor centre, to use an antiquated but expressive term, is a summation apparatus. That fact of itself precludes the grading of muscular activation from being based solely on number of motor units. With extensity-grading must be associated intensity-grading, i.e. grading, arrived at by summation, of the rate of discharge of the individual motor unit. Even in a reflex so simple as a spinal flexion twitch evoked by a single centripetal volley while some motoneurones are activated some are excited only subliminally [77, 80]. Again, in the flexion reflex under a tetanic afferent stimulus there results along with tetanic activation of some motoneurones subliminal excitation of others [52]. Further, it can be shown that the reflex tetanic activation can be made *maximal* in the sense that some of the reflexly driven muscle-fibres are driven at their full tetanic contraction, the proof of this being that a concurrent reflex via another afferent, although competent to drive them of itself, does in fact contract them no further [52, 56]. Now, subliminal central excitation, i.e. central excitation too weak to cause centrifugal discharge to the muscle, and maximal central excitation, i.e. excitation intense enough to cause centrifugal discharge maximally tetanizing the muscle-fibres, are the two extremes of the scale of excitation. That both these extremes are in evidence in the motoneurone pool of a reflexly activated muscle argues a wide range of graded reflex excitement. Reflex excitation exerts therefore upon the individual motoneurones degrees of excitation which differ widely from motoneurone to motoneurone.

It was shown by Adrian [2] that the frequency of firing of a receptor organ and its nerve-fibre increases *ceteris paribus* with increase of intensity of the stimulation. Later, Adrian and Bronk [10] on the one hand, and Denny-Brown [63] on the other, by different methods and independently, succeeded in observing the reflex firing of individual motor units. They observed it to be of various rates in different motor units firing at the same time in the same muscle.

Rates observed ranged from 6–7.5 per sec. in slow extensor muscles (Figs. 25, 27) and from 15 per sec. in the motor phrenic up to 60 and 80 per sec. (Fig. 4). Here, as with receptor-discharge, rate of firing indicates *ceteris paribus* degree of excitation. Thus in the phrenic the individual motor-fibre fires more rapidly with stronger inspiration [10]. With decerebrate soleus the isolated motor unit responds to increase of the contralateral stimulus by firing faster; under transient reflex inhibition its rate of firing slackens (Fig. 53) [63]. The different rates of firing among the motor units engaged in the same reflex indicate therefore that the reflex is operating on them with individually different degrees of excitation.

Among the rates of reflex firing some are below that required for full tetanization of their muscle-fibres. Since the rate of firing increases with increasing reflex excitation this adjustment of the degree of imperfect tetanization contributes to quantitative adjustment of the reflex contraction. It is convenient to designate as *subtetanus* [191] all tetanization which is imperfect and falls short of the rate at which mechanical fusion of the tetanus is complete, completeness meaning that no increase of frequency or strength of stimulus can increase the contraction tension further. Between rate of subtetanus and height of contraction tension a definite relation holds, and this has been determined in the case of regular rates of subtetanization for some of the muscles commonly employed in reflex observations (Cooper and Eccles) [57]. The relation follows an S-shaped curve (Fig. 60).

Along with tetanus, subtetanus obtains in the reflexly excited muscle. Some motoneurones will be firing at tetanic rates, others at subtetanic rates, and some not firing at all although under excitement; others, further, will not be firing because not under excitement at all. According to their state or grade of reflex excitation the engaged motoneurones are of three classes—'subliminals', 'subtetanics', and 'maximals'. Each of these classes serves the quantitative adjustment of the reflex contraction, and each somewhat in its own way. In the sub-

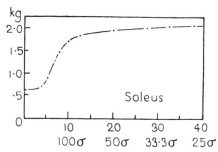

Fig. 60. Curve showing the effect of rate of stimulation on tetanus-tension of M. soleus. The values in sigmata under the rates are the intervals between stimuli at those rates.

tetanics the two modes of adjustment (1) change in number of units engaged and (2) change in intensity of activation of the individual unit, both take part to the full; but in the two others the latter change acts only indirectly and in so far as it can induce the former.

'*Subliminals*'. These may be regarded as the primary medium of recruitment. They mediate between activated centre and quiescent pool outside. The subliminal class is the seat of *addition latente* [189] and of the recruiting opening of the crossed extensor reflex. As 'fringe' [69] it recruits from the quiescent pool; back into that pool it sheds. Its relation to the supra-liminal field is sometimes illustrated under conditions strikingly simple [80, 191].

Two similar centripetal volleys are fired into the reflex centre in quick succession. Each volley when not following the other excites a reflex twitch indicating discharge of 13·8 per cent. of the motor units of the muscle. But when following on the other one volley adds a tension indicating 22·5 per cent. of the motor units, i.e. a subliminal fringe of 8·7 per cent. traceable to the precurrent volley was discharged by the second volley. Increasing the size of the volleys changed the numbers to 22·9 per cent. and 9·2 per cent. respectively. With further increase of the volleys the discharge effected by each singly became 34·4 per cent. but the subliminal fringe as revealable by the second volley had almost disappeared. The units which had been subliminals with the smaller volley had with the larger centripetal volley become supraliminals.

The *d'emblée* opening seen commonly in the spinal flexion reflex (Fig. 10) under direct faradic stimulation of a bared afferent nerve is not to be regarded as typical of 'natural' reflexes. The sudden outburst into full tetanic activity on the part of many of the motor units activated is in a sense 'artificial'. Cutaneous or proprioceptive stimuli are not easily imagined which will develop their effect rectangularly with the suddenness of a faradic current on an afferent nerve-trunk. The reflex excitement of a motor unit, even if it is to be high, commonly in natural reflexes rises gradually.

The effectiveness of the subliminal fringe as a liaison between reflexes which, although separately barely effective, co-operate with success for muscular effects exemplifies the subliminals as an initial basis for recruitment of reflex activity. Thus, limb stimuli seemingly ineffective become effective by turning the head, though this latter is likewise ineffective when alone [17].

Summation being additive presents also a subtraction counterpart, 'de-recruitment'. The slope of the post-stimulation termination of a reflex is, owing to after-discharge, commonly not abrupt. A fringe that has by summation been raised to supraliminal may persist supraliminally even after withdrawal of its original afferent stimulus if the concomitant afferent stimulus be sustained, 'sustained facilitation' (Eccles and Granit) [75]. In the decerebrate preparation the crossed extension reflex leaves behind it a temporary facilitation for the stretch reflex of the extensor muscle [122]. The final stage of activity in the centre, as its reflex subsides, must commonly be a state of subliminal excitation at the internuncial relays where those are involved. With 'natural' stimuli, e.g. skin pressure, the centripetal stream itself does not drop to zero with the abruptness of a faradic stimulus withdrawn, so that the post-stimulation phase is then still less abrupt than in the faradized-nerve form of the spinal flexion reflex. This latter therefore both at beginning and at ending presents artificiality.

As to the proportion of subliminals to supraliminals in the excited centre, there are instances where the *whole* central effect, in weak reflexes, may as regards a particular muscle be subliminal. Above, an instance was given of a subliminal fringe nearly half as extensive as the whole activated fraction.

In this instance, however, the values found for the fringe are artificially low. (1) The second stimulus following so closely must fall within the relative refractory phase of some of the afferent fibres just previously excited by the first single shock (Forbes) [89]. (2) The stimulus series being confined to two successive volleys, effective summation is more limited than where a longer serial iteration has play, as in the *addition latente* of the crossed extensor reflex.

Very large subliminal fringes have been observed with the decerebrate extension reflex (Eccles and Granit) [75] under interaction of weak tetanic stimuli with pairs of allied contralateral nerves as afferents. The labyrinth reflexes have large fringes [17] for the extensor muscles of the hind limb, and so also Rademaker's plantar reflex [63]. With these last two sources the degree of excitation at command seems predominantly of lower rather than of higher grade, e.g. subliminals, and slower subtetanics rather than quicker subtetanics and maximals. Reflex sources differ not only in extensity of centrifugal distribution, i.e. number of motor units they affect in a given motoneurone pool, but also in the intensity of distribution upon the pool, i.e. the intensity of influence on the individual motor unit. There are thus afferent sources of low-grade influence, e.g. labyrinthine on limb-extensors, which are nevertheless of wide extent in their muscular field, and others of high-grade influence but restricted extent, e.g. a dorsal digital on limb flexors. In the instance (p. 119) with two single-shock stimuli (flexion reflex) the fringe shrank relatively as the stimulus was strengthened. Exceptionally the spinal flexor (semitendinosus) responds maximally and *in toto*, so that all subliminals have been raised into maximals. Since, however, the reflex activates concurrently several synergic muscles, that does not say that the fringe is wanting altogether from the reflex.

In the accompanying chart (Fig. 61) suppose an afferent nerve purely excitatory for the muscle in question, and that a break-shock series stimulating it be reduced in strength with consequent decrease in number of its stimulated fibres the decrease being among the smaller of the fibres previously excited. The field

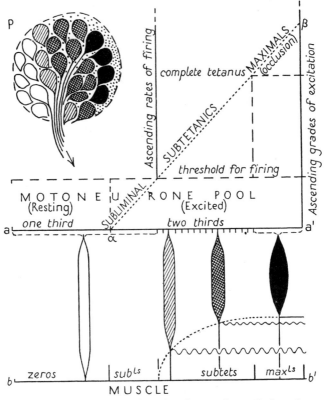

FIG. 61. Scheme of distribution of excitement in a reflexly active moto-neurone pool of a muscle. Grades of excitement plotted against numbers of motoneurones [abscissa *a a'*] and of motor-units [abscissa *b b'*]. *αβ* denotes excitements in active fraction of pool.

and density of the exciting central terminals are thus reduced. If we imagine this to reduce existing excitements by a given, say just subliminal amount, we may sample its effect on the various motor units along the scale of excitation of the chart. Subjected to this reduction the old subliminal fringe drops out altogether. The total excited field thus shrinks, i.e. the point *α* in the abscissa line *aa'* lies less far to the left. A new subliminal fringe is formed from lower 'subtetanics' which under the change drop to subliminal grade.

Conversely, if the stimulation of the afferent nerve be increased so as to heighten the number of excited fibres, especially adding those of smaller calibre, the field and density of the exciting central terminals are augmented. Fresh motoneurones are recruited from the quiescent 'zero' field. If now we suppose the increase of excitation such as to enhance existing excitements by a just subliminal amount, the existing subliminal fringe then disappears, being lifted into the subtetanic levels. The field of excitement is larger and the amount of muscular contraction is increased.

The subtetanics. Here in each unit the integrated tension of contraction falls variously short of full tetanic. The shortage is of course greater the slower the wave succession. The scale of grading becomes progressively less open as full tetanus is approached. A given increment of frequency of firing yields less increment of contraction tension in proportion as the frequency of firing is already high, until at last it yields no increase at all (occlusion) [52]. The frequency in some subtetanics can be lower than 10 per sec., though 60 per sec. be required for full tetanus. What percentage of the total of the engaged motor units in a given reflex may be driven subtetanically is difficult to ascertain. In the weak postural and crossed reflexes (decerebrate) of soleus search for separately registrable motor units not rarely fails to discover a single motor unit firing otherwise than in subtetanus. A slight increase in the contralateral stimulus can be observed to cause, along with acceleration of one unit, the entrance into action of one or more fresh ones; or conversely, slight weakening of the stimulus may bring cessation of the slower of the two units with slackening of the beat of the faster one. The change observed is predominantly consensual. This suggests that the limits of difference at any one time are not extreme.

Here again adjustment of amount of contraction includes adjustment both of the number of contracting units and of degree of contraction of the individual unit, i.e. proceeds by extensity and intensity. Subtetanic activation preponderates characteristically in the opening phase [10] of spinal and decerebrate reflexes, especially under 'natural' stimuli; also in the terminal phase as the reflex wanes away. If in the chart a small change of excitation be supposed, and its effect be sampled on various individuals of the subtetanic class, it is seen to adjust contraction by adjusting the rate of subtetanus. Further, if the change be increase, some subtetanics rise into, and so recruit, the 'maximals' class; if decrease, some degrade to subliminals, and some maximals become subtetanics.

Subtetanic contraction is tremulous. With a 'power' unit like that of gastrocnemius, which averages a contraction twitch of (cat) some 8 g. [78], its tremulous contraction, e.g. at 20 per sec. or less, must threaten the steadiness of the whole muscle. But this defect is lessened by the various subtetanized units being out of phase one with another. Inherent also in the operation of the subtetanized motor units is some waste of work, a waste which has been examined quantitatively by Bronk [33].

The maximals. In this group each unit yields full contraction, hence all additional excitement lays aside its mechanical equivalent, and all reduction of excitement short of removal of its units from the group altogether makes, as regards contraction-value, no difference. Each motor unit added to the group means increase on previous contraction and each removed from it means contraction lessened. In this group therefore adjustment of contraction is purely by extensity, i.e. by adjustment of number of units. This group accounts mainly for the occlusion of contraction which characteristically and commonly results under concurrence of spinal reflexes activating the same muscle (Fig. 11).

In weak reflexes, for instance in weak postural reflexes, there may be no maximals at all. The maximals grow prominent with strengthening of the reflex. In a strong reflex there may be none but 'maximals' in the entire motoneurone pool of a muscle [51, 52] as driven in laboratory experiment. Thus there is in the relation between increase of reflex contraction and increase of reflex stimulation some resemblance to the approximately logarithmic ratio between increment of sensation and increment of stimulus. The difference of contraction which a given increase or decrease of excitation occasions in a motor unit is less according as that unit already lies high in the scale of excited states; once the unit is in the maximals increment of excitation causes no difference of contraction tension at all. A maximally run unit is *ceteris paribus* more economical than a subtetanic, since the contraction tension is maintained at relatively smaller expenditure of energy.

The motor centre even at its spinal simplest is more than a mere passive relay forwarding impulses on their way out to their muscle. It is an instrument which always actively summates the excitatory effects of its incoming impulses; on that quantitative basis it starts new impulses, and quantitatively adjusts the reflex contraction. Thus is varied the number of motoneurones engaged, and thus a whole scale of grades of excitement are exerted on the individual motoneurone.

Under full natural conditions the grading does not end with that. We have then to envisage the further interplay between the graded excitation and graded inhibition coincident concurrently on the centre.

Quantitative course of a simple reflex.

In the course of a reflex a given motoneurone climbs and then descends the scale of excitements [10]. The rate of discharge of the individual motor unit alters during the course of the reflex. An outstanding instance is the progressive increase of rate accompanying the opening phase of many spinal and decerebrate reflexes, especially when provoked by natural stimuli. The rate of firing of the unit is found to ascend the subtetanic scale and enter, it may be, 'maximal' grade (60 per sec.) in the course, it may be, of some 5 sec.; thus, in the decerebrate extensor reflex from a pinch of the opposite foot. In the spinal flexion reflex under a mechanical skin stimulus a similar course is run; the divergence which is so striking between this flexion reflex and the crossed extension reflex, as regards their opening phases when evoked by tetanization of a bared afferent nerve, largely disappears when a mechanical skin stimulus is used.

The abrupt onset of contraction of the spinal flexion reflex in response to a tetanizing current applied to the bared afferent nerve occurs by reason of the motor units entering into their full activity at once, in accord with the form of the centripetal stream received from the afferent nerve; in this latter the 'rectangular' stimulus excites its full measure of fibres at once and continues to do so at the experimentally imposed tetanizing rate. The *d'emblée* opening of the reflex response is thus artificial in the sense that it can hardly occur under 'natural' stimuli. But its occurrence shows that the reflex discharge conforms in this case fairly faithfully in quantitative course to the centripetal impulse-stream evoking it. The reflex contraction as evoked by a tetanizing current is sometimes almost indistinguishable from the tetanic contraction to a stimulus of like rate applied to the motor-nerve [117].

The *d'emblée* opening of the myogram of the spinal flexion reflex is sometimes more rectangular than even its standard of comparison, the motor tetanus. Where the interval between the successive break-shocks allows the tracing of the successive steps of the contraction response, the second step (response to second centripetal volley) may then be found to be much smaller than its predecessor [190]. The first step of the ascent of tension is relatively high to the next succeeding. This gives an abrupt turn from the ascent to the plateau accentuating further the *d'emblée* character. This accentuation of the *d'emblée* form is a still further departure from the 'natural', being an outcome of artificial admixture of inhibition and excitation. Yet although artificial, it is none the less the correct product of an efficiently working reflex centre of simple type dealing faithfully with an artificial form of stimulus. It is a correct answer, so to say, to an improper or wrong question.

On the other hand, the crossed extensor reflex presents commonly the recruiting commencement (p. 63) which is the very opposite of the *d'emblée*, and yet its recruitment as usually obtained appears again to be an artefact. The recruitment is very variable in its progress; sometimes it proceeds extremely slowly. It too seems to represent a conflict between inhibition and excitation, the former obstructing the very outset of the latter. In its extreme form this reflex result assumes a character which is obviously unnatural. Here the unnatural character of the stimulation, namely, wholesale excitation of the admixed fibres of a large afferent nerve-trunk, is again to be held responsible; a thoroughly artificial stimulus admixing excitation and inhibition grossly and causing an unnatural muscular result.

The denial of normal co-ordination to these reflex responses, which after all are orderly, may seem unwarranted. The suggestion is, however, not that they are wholly inco-ordinate. The 'centre' subjects to co-ordination whatever passes through it, i.e. whatever reflex stream it deals with. In other words every motor discharge it delivers, every muscular contraction it produces, is in so far a co-ordinated product. It is, in a sense, true to say that every reflex discharge is co-ordinate; and such assertion has the merit of clearly recognizing that reflex co-ordination has its degrees.

The submission to the spinal 'centre' of abnormal and 'artificially' consorted streams of centripetal impulses, e.g. under naked nerve faradization, does not result in wholly 'inco-ordinate' contraction. The 'jet' reflex, the 'reversal' responses, 'rebounds', the hesitating recruitment of some extensor reflexes and so on, are not inco-ordinate reflexes although not examples of normal co-ordination. Responses manufactured by elementary co-ordination from thoroughly abnormal ingredient stimuli are faulty, but they teach certain facts about elementary co-ordination, perhaps, peculiarly well.

At the same time it is to be remembered that 'recruitment' does appear under 'natural' stimulation, and not only as the result of the centripetal stream itself under a 'natural' stimulus having an 'increasing' opening. That alone does not account for the whole recruitment, because its characteristic course disappears on deafferenting the reacting muscle (p. 136), e.g. in Philippson's reflex.

Philippson's reflex as originally observed was extension on one knee in the chronic spinal dog evoked by passive flexion of the other. It was shown subsequently that it can be well obtained in the acute decerebrate preparation [177]. In the manipulation the pressure exerted on the skin is not an essential part of the stimulus. The reflex is of proprioceptive source, for it is found [177] to be obtainable in the decerebrate preparation with the vasto-crureus nerve only remaining on one side and the motor-nerve to vasto-crureus only on the other. In the cat it operates the crossed soleus as well as the vasto-crureus.

The spinal reflex excited in tibialis anticus by a pressure applied to a digit shows a gradual opening; contraction and action-currents increase progressively, even after a spring clip quickly attached. The centripetal flow itself, to judge from Adrian's observations, grows in rate and volume. The reflex centre's discharge follows this course of inflow sufficiently faithfully for the muscular contraction broadly to correspond with it.

Again, the reflex contraction from the spring clip left in position quite quickly dwindles (acute spinal preparation), although in the same experiment faradic stimulation of an adjacent plantar nerve filament maintains a plateau-contraction of about the same height with little decline for a longer period. Cessation of the digital pinch is followed by reflex discharge for much longer than is cessation of the faradic stimulus of the bared nerve. The above three features distinguishing the form of the 'spinal' flexor discharge evoked by a 'pinch' from that by a faradized afferent nerve, all seem traceable to the difference in volume and course of the centripetal impulse-stream obtaining for the two. The relatively gradual opening and decline of such a 'natural' reflex, involving and releasing its motor units smoothly, bears resemblance in quantitative course to the central discharge, e.g. into an inspiratory muscle, under normal rhythmic activation.

Plurimuscular combination in the reflex.

In dealing with the overlapping and gradual engagement of the motoneurones in a reflex it was simpler to treat the motoneurone pool as that of a single muscle. But a reflex always in fact engages more than one muscle. The 'motor centre' is plurimuscular. Thus, in the protective reflex of flexion, in response to harmful stimulation of the foot, flexors of hip, knee, and ankle are activated together. The advantage for the effect in view is obvious. On close examination a stimulus applied to the focal area [178] of the receptive field of the reflex excites practically synchronously the main flexors of hip and knee and ankle. With increase of stimulus and reflex the degree of engagement extends in each muscle, though not necessarily *pari passu* in all [58]. With electrical stimuli of the bared afferent nerves the result is similar, except that the reflex result is less homogeneous, the protective flexion may be mixed with flexion-phase of step, with ipselateral extension, &c.

The quantitative adjustment of the reflex contraction involves therefore co-adjustment in the motoneurone pools of several muscles. In great part this, in a simple spinal reflex, seems referable to actual central distribution of the afferent nerve-fibres. The afferent fibre branches intraspinally and its central terminals have plurimuscular distribution, in the sense that indirectly or directly they serve to excite motoneurones of several synergic muscles. The co-adjustment of the synergic muscles is also helped by proprioceptive reflexes initiated by and from the active muscles themselves. Thus, the reflex combination of synergic muscles, e.g. of one limb-flexor with another, is reinforced by the proprioceptive reflex of one flexor exciting another flexor. The active contraction of a flexor, especially against resistance, evokes through proprioceptors of that flexor muscle reflex activation of other flexors [53, 55]. Thus, contraction of tibialis anticus (ankle flexor) evokes reflexly a contraction of sartorius (knee and hip flexor). The stretch reflex from passive stretch evoked in the knee-extensor, vastus internus, spreads its excitatory effect to the synergic ankle-extensor, soleus [63]. The 'lengthening' reaction of one vasto-crureus has as concomitant an active postural contraction of the other vasto-crureus [177].

The executant musculature itself thus provides a reflex means of supporting or reinforcing the co-operation of flexors with flexors, extensors with extensors, &c. The proprioceptors of reacting muscles operate reflexly upon other muscles of near functional relation to themselves. Active contraction (including active stretch) and passive stretch in the reacting muscles are stimuli for reflexes influencing other muscles, and the reflex influence so exerted is on some muscles excitatory and on others inhibitory [55, 62]; it is largely reciprocally distributed, knitting synergists together.

RECIPROCAL INNERVATION

Reflexes finding expression in the skeletal musculature have a field inhibitory as well as excitatory; and the distribution of the central process is for inhibition plurimuscular as it is for excitation. In the nociceptive reflex of the hind limb the inhibitory side of the reflex has been observed to include the following muscles [178]: vasti, crureus, rectus femoris, gastrocnemius, soleus, semimembranosus, biceps femoris (posterior portion), quadratus femoris, adductor magnus (a part of), adductor minor.

The inhibitory central field commonly includes the motoneurone pools of muscles directly antagonistic to those excited (reciprocal innervation). Intraspinal branching of the afferent root-fibres probably goes far to secure this. The arrangement would then be much as though the scheme which in Astacus is peripheral and efferent to the antagonistic muscles of the claw were here inverted and afferent and distributed centrally to antagonistic motoneurones. If so it would seem that co-operative contraction of such directly antagonistic muscles will always involve admixture of inhibition with excitation.

The field which is excitatory engages motoneurones overlapped by inhibitory fields of other reflexes; so also the inhibitory field overlaps the excitatory of other reflexes. Opposition between central excitation and central inhibition is quantitative; a grading of reflex activation of a muscle is thus obtainable not only by grading of excitation but also by grading of inhibition. When two afferents, one excitatory the other inhibitory, for a given muscle are concurrently stimulated, adjustment of the amount of resultant contraction is possible over a wide range by adjusting the strength of stimulation of either or of both the nerves (Fig. 62).

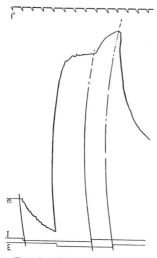

FIG. 62. Algebraic summation of excitatory and inhibitory reflexes on the same muscle, decerebrate vasto-crureus. Upper signal *I* marks period of stimulation by a break-shock series at 30 per sec. of the ipselateral peroneal afferent. Lower signal *E* marks similar stimulation of the contralateral popliteal afferent.

The resultant contraction taken in its aggregate effect upon the muscle exhibits a compromise between the two opposed effects, an 'algebraical summation' of them [174]. The inhibitory subtraction from the excitatory field is in fact composed of effects taking place in the units of the field as a group in one or both of two ways: (a) total suppression of the centrifugal discharge of the motoneurone with corresponding relaxation of the corresponding muscle-fibres, (b) slackening of the tetanic or subtetanic discharge of the motoneurone with partial relaxation of the corresponding muscle-fibres (see Fig. 61). A twitch reflex can similarly be diminished by adjusting the strength of a single-shock inhibitory volley. In this instance the grading is wholly by variation of the number of motor units suppressed.

Reflex inhibition can grade the amplitude of rhythmic reflexes, e.g. spinal stepping; but it has never been observed to alter the rate of rhythm of 'scratching', although it can readily suppress the scratching altogether.

In respect to reciprocal innervation distinction has to be drawn between antagonists and pseud-antagonists. A muscle which by fixing a joint enhances the effect of another muscle crossing that joint to act on a further one, is said to be the latter muscle's pseud-antagonist. In simple reflex flexion of the knee *semitendinosus*, a knee flexor, contracts, while *vasto-crureus*, the knee-extensor, relaxes (reciprocal innervation). But at hip semitendinosus is an extensor, and the reflex taxis throws it and the hip flexors into contraction together. The hip flexors by preventing hip-extension antagonize semitendinosus in its action at the hip but enhance it as a flexor of the knee. Similarly, gastrocnemius has at ankle a true antagonist in tibialis anticus, and reciprocal innervation holds between them; but at knee gastrocnemius has a pseud-antagonist in vasto-crureus, and reflex co-contraction obtains between them. That gastrocnemius itself, a double-joint muscle, crosses the flexor aspect of the knee makes it, even when passive and still more so when active, a 'muscular ligament' enabling the quadriceps extensor of the knee to extend powerfully not only the knee but the ankle. Pseud-antagonism is really a form of synergism and reflex co-ordination deals with it as with other synergism not by reciprocal innervation but by co-contraction.

Examination of 'reciprocal innervation' by the myograph introduces the artificial conditions that contraction of one antagonist, e.g. the shortening of the 'prime mover', no longer pulls on the opponent, e.g. no longer exerts stretch of it, the muscles for attachment to the myograph being freed from their natural insertions. Taking as instance the reflex flexion of knee evoked by a nociceptive stimulus applied to the foot in the decerebrate preparation; the contraction of the knee-flexor is then accompanied by the well-known inhibitory relaxation of the knee-extensor as examined by the myograph. If, however, the muscles were still attached to the leg the flexor's action would entail pull upon the extensor, and such pull is the adequate stimulus for the stretch reflex of the extensor. The reciprocal inhibition of the extensor will then be faced by an access of reflex excitation from the stretch. Under the artificially simplified conditions of the myographic examination this excitation is not present. There is also the contingency of a 'lengthening reaction' in the pulled extensor (autogenous inhibition). The reciprocal inhibition may be thought of as itself too potent to allow the further stretch to operate reflexly. But such a point cannot be discounted in the consideration of co-ordination until direct experimental evidence has shown neglect of it to be permissible.

With the antagonists at the ankle Graham Brown [41] has observed that with the two opposed muscles, detached and separately recording their contractions isotonically against light resistance (10 grm.) and operated reflexly by successive stimuli in a series of graded strengths, the active shortening of the one muscle added to the relaxation-lengthening of the other sum for each observation of the series to the same figure throughout the series. The percentage contraction of the one runs a course which is in percentage of the total just converse to that of the inhibitory relaxation of the other. Did this represent a universal rule it would be possible to assess inco-ordination by departure from it. No 'double-joint' head of a muscle consists of fibres of the 'slow' contraction type, and the 'rapid' head of a muscle lies superficial. Hence each 'slow' muscle (knee, ankle, shoulder, elbow) has attached to its tendon a 'quick' muscle often of double-joint disposition. The functional significance of 'slow' muscle has been discussed earlier (pp. 57–60, 78).

There is, further, 'double reciprocal innervation' [175] where a pair of opponent muscles are under the influence of two concurrent stimuli each of which treats the antagonistic muscles on the reciprocal plan but is itself individually opposed to the other stimulus in the direction of its influence on those muscles. Reciprocal innervation need not imply that of two antagonist muscles both cannot be in contraction at the same time; rather it implies that they are. Its characteristic is that increase of contraction in one member of the paired set goes with decrease of contraction in the other. But cases occur where in neither of the two antagonists does outward change of contraction ensue although the innervation is changing. A peculiarly simple type instance of this is that of the eye, where a fixated object approaches along the line of vision of one eye. Unchanging conjugate deviation is then concurrent with increasing convergence, the former activating, e.g. lateral rectus, the latter medial rectus. Reciprocal innervation obtains for these muscles [156, 157], and thus for the medial rectus of the unmoved eye increasing excitation from one source (convergence) combines with balanced inhibition from the other source.

The inhibitory effect on antagonists (i.e. on the 'half-centres' of Graham Brown) which assures reciprocal innervation seems a central disposition as direct as that securing excitation. But this arrangement is enlarged and reinforced by proprioceptive reflexes interacting between, e.g. limb muscles (p. 129). Thus, severance of the hamstring nerve (dog, cat) heightens the reflex contraction of its antagonist muscle, quadriceps [154, 155]; weak stimulation of that nerve inhibits knee-jerk and knee-tonus [155, 168]. Active contraction of the hamstring muscles gives reflex inhibition of quadriceps [55, 154]: stretching or kneading of semimembranosus gives reflex inhibition of knee-jerk [154]: stretching of posterior biceps gives reflex inhibition of vasto-crureus stretch reflex [120]. A stretch in one extensor, causing a 'lengthening reaction' in it, causes inhibition of a stretch reflex present in another extensor [62].

Reciprocal innervations occur in reflex co-ordination of *symmetrical* right and left muscles as pairs (Fig. 63); for instance, in the knee-extensors or the hip flexors reflexly operated from limb afferents of either hind limb [179]. Here the crossed effect which is the reciprocal of the ipselateral involves an internuncial neurone, and is less stable, i.e. more easily disturbed by competitive reflexes, than in reciprocal innervation of true antagonists. So also with the sternomastoids as reflexly operated by cervical afferents. The medial and lateral eyeball recti exhibit reciprocal innervation in reflex vestibular nystagmus [73, 112, 113]; also under cortical stimulation directing the gaze [157], and under willed direction of it [1]. The rhythmic reflexes of the 'scratch' and of stepping exhibit 'reciprocal innervation' in their prime movers at ankle, and probably at other joints.

'Double reciprocal innervation' provides good instances of the concurrent presence of reflex excitation in muscles of opposed effect, the admixture of excitation and inhibition being

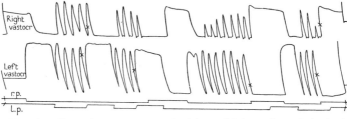

FIG. 63. Decerebrate vasto-crurei, right and left; reciprocal rhythmic contractions and inhibitory relaxations evoked in the right and left muscles by concurrent faradization of the right and left peroneal nerves (afferent).

here more normally distributed than under stimulation of a single afferent. Quantitative estimation of an inhibitory reflex has to reckon with the fact that inhibition can only document itself against excitement, e.g. as relaxation of contraction. Of a central field of inhibition that portion if any which corresponds with unexcited portions of, for instance, a reflexly reacting motoneurone pool will not give any evidence of its existence by effect on the reflex contraction. This is the 'ineffective inhibition' of Graham Brown [39]. With weak inhibition and weak excitation exerted concurrently on the same motoneurone pool each may affect motoneurones unaffected by the other [59], and there will in so far be no evidence of the weak inhibition. With strong stimulation, however, of even small afferent nerves the central inhibition they induce can cover fractions of the motor centre larger than those which the excitatory field of the afferent correspondingly stimulated can attain [59]. When the reciprocal extensor inhibition adjunct to a constant submaximal flexion reflex is pitted against extensor tonic reflexes of different magnitudes the inhibitory relaxations are greater the greater the extensor contraction. Isotonically registered the relaxation removes at each assay approximately the same proportion of the several contractions offered [40, 41]. There are therefore cases where the grade of inhibition, compounded both of numbers and intensities of units though it be, is, when sampled in larger and larger pieces, found spread evenly throughout a great range of excitation.

'Co-contraction' is a frequent normal feature of reflex 'fixation' of joints, e.g. in the supporting reaction of the fore-limbs [143, 145, 153]. In standing the apex of the limb is fixated by synergic contraction of antagonists. The mutual co-ordination of antagonists at more proximal joints also is in postural fixation, e.g. standing, quite other than in movements, in which latter reciprocal innervation prevails. Sharp distinction between the two forms of co-ordination, reciprocal innervation and co-contraction, is difficult in the case of double-joint muscles, and especially in those of opposed effect on their two joints respectively, e.g. rectus femoris a flexor at hip and an extensor at knee; contraction here of the muscle isolated for the myograph may be equivocal in significance as between its action as a prime mover or a fixator. Moreover, postural action occurs not merely in the intervals between movements but commonly is concurrently commingled with them (Cobb).

SPEED OF MOVEMENT

With isotonic records of reflex contraction the rate of shortening, i.e. the speed of movement, increases, other things equal, with intensity of the reflex stimulation. Isometric observations are of course less suitable for study of movement; in them tension, so to say, replaces movement.

A remarkable alteration as to speed of movement of the reflexly reacting muscle is observed after severance of the afferent nerves of the muscle itself [177] in the case of extensor muscles. To examine this it is needful to eschew isometry and to avoid using as reflex stimulus the faradization of a bared afferent nerve, this latter because the recruiting opening of the extensor reflex then obtained is largely traceable to and complicated by conflict of reflex excitation with inhibition owing to admixture of inhibitory with excitatory afferents in the afferent nerve-trunk stimulated. The complication is avoided by using for evoking, e.g. the crossed extensor reflex, a natural stimulus, namely passive flexion of the opposite knee [177]. The passive flexion is exerted against the postural extension of the knee maintained by a tonic vasto-crureus, which has been preserved as the only sentient structure in the limb, e.g. right. The preparation is decerebrate, and the other limb, i.e. left, similarly prepared, is, making use of its plasticity of posture, set with some flexion at knee. Passive flexion of the extended right knee is then made; it excites reflex inhibition of its own vasto-crureus accompanied by reflex contraction of the contralateral vasto-crureus at the left knee. The extension movement executed by this latter proceeds with a characteristic unabrupt deliberateness and passes smoothly over into a maintained posture without undue haste or overshoot from momentum. This reaction, when repeated with the one difference of condition that the contralateral, i.e. left extensor, has been deafferented, is executed obviously differently from before by that muscle, i.e. by left vasto-crureus; the movement originally smooth and deliberate has become an abrupt rush of sudden contraction, with development of momentum, and usually of exaggerated amplitude (Fig. 64). In the muscle with its afferents intact the course and speed of its reflex contraction is controlled by some 'braking' action attributable to proprioceptives of the contracting muscle itself. The cutting of these entailed therefore a loss of some restraint which they exerted reflexly upon their own muscle during its contraction. It appears therefore that an extensor muscle, when contracting in adjustment of posture, 'brakes' its own speed of movement or tantamountly restrains its own rate of development of tension, and does this by reflexly controlling itself through some of its own proprioceptives (autogenous inhibition).

There are several possible ways in which this might be effected. The reflex contraction of a muscle is a partial contraction, and when with its afferents intact it partially contracts, and especially when it is allowed to shorten it replaces, in so far as proprioceptive stimulation is concerned, passive tension by active tension. A restricted extent of this latter may relieve a considerably larger extent of the former; the muscle as it contracts would thus reduce a myotatic reinforcement. Severance of the afferents of the contracting muscle would bring loss both of myotatic reinforcement and of this means of reducing it were it present. On the other hand, among the proprioceptives of the extensor muscles are some which can reflexly inhibit the muscle's own contraction [170], e.g. the lengthening reaction. The reflex contraction may excite these. The contraction of the knee-jerk

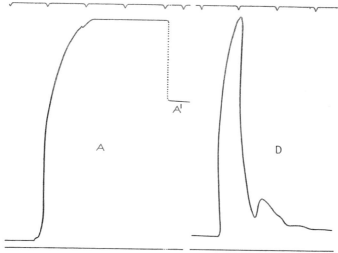

FIG. 64. Decerebrate vasto-crureus; reflex response to passive flexion of the contralateral knee before (A) and (D) after [48 days] severance of the afferent nerve-roots of the responding vasto-crureus muscle. A' continuance of A, 60 seconds later. Isotonic myograph. Time, 1 sec.

can excite from the muscle some centripetal impulses which are inhibitory of limb-extensors [62].

The muscle's reflex response to an extraneous excitation brings in factors of co-ordination traceable to the proprioceptors of the muscle itself. These autogenous factors are of two kinds, one exerting on the motoneurones of their own muscle excitatory influence, the other inhibitory. During their co-operation they interact with various grades of result. The 'self-braking' action as an attribute of normal extensor reflex response thus finds its basis. In Fig. 64 the course of the undeafferented extensor muscle's contraction under the 'natural' stimulus shows an evident 'recruiting' opening, though of less accentuated type than is common when the crossed extensor reflex is operated by the 'unnatural' stimulation of a faradic series applied to a naked afferent nerve-trunk. In this latter case the slowly progressive recruitment was regarded (pp. 67, 126) as meaning a struggle between admixed excitation and inhibition. The milder restraint and quicker smooth recruitment under the 'natural' stimulus, though partly due to peripheral afferent recruitment, indicates a normal and natural co-operation of excitation and inhibition which, since it disappears (Fig. 64) when the muscle is deafferented, is an autogenous reflex product of the muscle itself and in so far is intrinsically operated by it.

The explosive rush and momentum characterizing the effect of deafferenting the executant muscles in these low-level extensor reflexes have their counterpart in the ataxy of tabes, and in similar features attaching even more strikingly to movements of a completely deafferented limb [191] acting under operation of the 'will'. The resemblance of co-ordinative defect in the two indicates that the self-restraint observable in the decerebrate extensor reflex and there abrogated by destruction of the extensor muscle's own proprioceptives plays its part too in the muscular behaviour under the will, for there too it is abrogated by deafferenting the executant muscles.

TREMOR

With faradic series as stimuli applied to bared afferent nerves a tremor occurs in the reflex contraction corresponding in frequency with that of the stimulus series unless that frequency is above a certain rate. This may occur with frequencies as high even as 95 a second. It is a feature traceable to the artificial stimulation employed. It results from the synchronism of the rhythm of excitation which these artificial stimuli impose directly on the afferent nerve-fibres, a synchronism to which natural stimuli applied to specific receptors offer little counterpart. The stimulation tremor does not arise to equal extent in all reflexes; under the same rate of serial stimulation there is much difference between the spinal flexor reflex and the crossed extensor reflex [116]. In the latter the centripetal impulse volley, acting through an internuncial relay as it does, tends to temporal spread in its effect on the motoneurone and its primary rhythm is confused and smothered both in myograph and galvanometer at lower frequencies than in the flexor reflex. The prominence of stimulus rhythm in the decerebrate extensor reflex is favoured (Fig. 65) by deafferenting the muscle [177], the smothering by secondary waves is therefore in part at least a proprioceptive reaction arising in the reacting muscle itself; that is, the contraction is steadied by means of a regulated

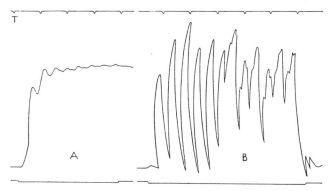

FIG. 65. Decerebrate vasto-crureus; crossed reflex excited by a series of break-shocks at 8 per sec. to the afferent popliteal nerve. *A*, normal muscle; *B*, fellow muscle deafferented 82 days. Time, 0·25 sec.

proprioceptive process taking origin in the reacting muscle itself.

The rhythm of an inhibitory stimulus can also make itself evident in a reflex contraction [97, 171]. This is seen especially where the inhibition is relatively weak, e.g. the same inhibitory stimulus which will smoothly relax the weakly rigid knee-extensor will against the strongly rigid produce a partial and tremulous relaxation—the rate of tremor being that of the inhibitory stimulus.

The contraction of decerebrate rigidity, enduring hour after hour as it will, is not, when minutely examined by the isotonic myograph, perfectly steady. During gradual increase or decrease it presents little steps of shortening or lengthening of the muscle. The tremor of its subtetanic units is obviated by their asynchronism. Gross clonus is easily developed from it, in the manner described above (p. 61, Fig. 29).

DIRECTION OF MOVEMENT; ORIENTATION OF POSTURE

For correctness of reflex co-ordination an acid test is whether the act duly attains its end. To apply this test the end must of course be known; and in some cases we know it sufficiently. When a fly alighting on the bulbo-spinal cat's pinna excites and is flicked off by the pinna reflex we may suppose that the movement has met its purpose. Again, when the spinal limb's flexion reflex, evoked by taking hold of or fixing a clip to the foot, succeeds through this-and-that way struggling in freeing the foot or flinging off the clip, the co-ordination can be judged as adequate for its end. But as to whether a knee-jerk is duly co-ordinate or not we have no criterion of 'end' to apply. Clue to 'aim' of a reflex strengthens with complexity of the reflex [182]. A gain secured by the plurimuscular co-operation inherent in reflexes is finer adjustment of direction of movement or of orientation of posture. Hence, refined evidence for assessing reflex co-ordination can be expected where *direction* of reflex movement can be judged as to rightness. This is especially possible where reflexes exhibit 'local sign' [162], i.e. where the reflex movement is specifically orientated in relation to the position of the peripheral stimulus.

The scratch reflex adjusts the direction of the hind foot so as to reach this or that point in an area of skin covering the side of the neck, chest, and flank, and extending from the ear to the loin. As a spinal reflex it can activate many muscles at a time, e.g. 36 have been observed. It combines alternating movement and steady posture; its posture coexisting with its movement. There is the rhythmic scratching movement involving digits, ankle, knee, and hip: there is further the postural flexion of the limb as a whole, and steady incurvation of the body with neck deviated and head partly turned back for the foot more readily to reach it. In the chronic 'spinal' dog the postural direction of the scratching limb noticeably follows the location of the stimulus in the receptive field; the scratching foot attains rarely, it is true, the actual locus of the stimulus. Deafferentation of the scratching limb [167] in the chronic spinal dog does not obviously impair the rhythmic movement and actually favours the ease of elicitation of the reflex; but it does impair the orientation of the reflex to local sign. The foot misses the seat of stimulation more widely. In the *acute* spinal preparation, e.g. in the decapitated cat, even without deafferentation, the misdirection of the scratching foot is often gross; and this is not wholly from loss of concomitant posture in the neck and head, for the scratching foot may operate in the air quite out of range of positions the receptive field could ever occupy. This impairment of orientation to 'local sign' contrasts with the slightness of impairment of the rhythmic movement itself; rate of rhythm is not altered nor its extent. In the decerebrate preparation the scratch reflex is less easily evoked than in the decapitate, but when one hind limb has been deafferented the reflex is more easily evoked from that limb, but exhibits the grosser lack of orientation to 'local sign'; so similarly in the chronic spinal dog. The inference is less that the afferents of the scratching limb supply guidance for the direction of its movements in accordance with 'local sign', than that that direction demands a more normal state of the limb-muscle centres in respect of balance, and especially of postural balance, e.g. between flexors and extensors, than the spinal or decerebrate preparation provides. That this defect is increased by deafferenting the limb-muscles is to be expected. It gives shrewd indication of the extent to which the execution of even a conscious act must be based upon, and therefore at the mercy of, automatic and proprioceptive co-ordination of bulbospinal level.

PHASES AND TURNING-POINTS; RHYTHMIC REFLEXES

The normal transition from one reflex to another presents a problem in reflex taxis. In the laboratory the experimentally isolated reflex is brought to conclusion by withdrawal of some singly operating stimulus. This procedure bears little resemblance to natural conditions where commonly many stimuli are at work together and each dominant one treads on the heel of a previously dominant; there reflex sequence is obtained against a background far from quiescent or unoccupied; and yet that sequence proceeds without confusion. Pattern succeeds pattern. The isolated reflex observed in the laboratory against a background of quiescence does not usually subside immediately on cessation of its stimulus. It has after-discharge. That after-discharge is, however, little resistent to inhibition. A new incoming reflex, opposed in direction to its predecessor, can remove any hampering or blocking after-discharge by the reciprocal inhibition which is part of itself (p. 129); just as, conversely, its excitation breaks through inhibitory after-action, which latter can be as marked as is excitatory after-discharge.

Sequence of reflexes is sometimes secured by the first reflex bringing about application of a stimulus which then excites a second reflex, and so on. Such is the restimulation of the scratch reflex by itself [168], and the self-restimulation of the jaw reflex [183]. Such also are 'chain-reflexes'. Again, with a sequence or train of allied reflexes there can be lowering of the threshold of each succeeding reflex by means of one just preceding it, e.g. in the scratch reflex by the spur-wheel or by a parasite travelling the receptive surface [167]. There the central subliminal response to the earlier stimulus facilitates response to the ensuing (positive successive induction) [168]. Conversely, a reflex, e.g. extension, may be favoured by precurrence of an opposite reflex of flexion (negative successive induction) [165, 168]. In this connexion interest attached to 'rebound' as a possible liaison [183] between successive phases of reflexes of alternating direction. But the artificial character of the stimulations under which rebounds occur [94] makes their interpretation for co-ordination difficult, although they do operate in some 'alternating' reflexes, e.g. reflex biting [183].

'Alternating' [168] reflexes have the feature that the direction of movement holding for a phase in one sense is followed by a phase of opposite direction and this in turn by reversion to the earlier phase, and so on, the alternation proceeding under continuance of the same unaltered stimulus. Some of the alternating reflexes are of irregular alternation, e.g. the release reflex of the foot, the pinna reflex. A number of them are, however, regularly rhythmic, e.g. stepping, the scratch reflex, the shake reflex of the body, the shake reflex of the head, the to-and-fro snout reflex, biting reflex of lower jaw [22, 183]. In these the movement proves to be not merely the alternate contraction and relaxation of a single prime mover or set of such; it is operated by alternate contraction of two opposed sets of prime movers, contraction in the one alternating with contraction in the other.

The problem is how, under continuance of unaltered stimulation, does the initial contraction, e.g. of the flexor, instead of persisting during the maintained stimulus, die out despite that stimulus, and why, as it does so, does contraction of the extensor occur in its stead, again then to give way to flexion, and so on? There is still much to learn about this, but certain points have interest and bearing.

(1) In the successive phases of the alternation (stepping, scratch) 'reciprocal innervation' obtains, i.e. while the flexors

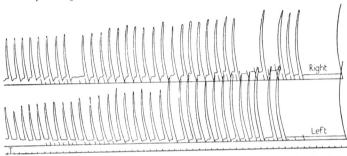

Fig. 66. Stepping movements at the ankles right and left (cat) arising under deep ether-chloroform narcosis, and becoming more ample as the depth of narcosis decreased, until they suddenly ceased. Time, 1 sec.

contract the extensors relax, and vice versa; sometimes a relaxation phase shows complete absence of motor discharges.

(2) The rhythm of alternation persists after deafferentation of the entire limb exhibiting the rhythm, e.g. scratch, step [37, 167, 178]. The 'spinal' limb 'steps' under a depth of narcosis which precludes reflex response to stimulation of the afferent nerves of the limb [37] (Fig. 66). The turning-point in these cases must be purely centrally operated.

(3) With a freshly made spinal severance at the last thoracic segment serving as stimulus a regular stepping of the hind limb ensues even when both hind limbs have been deafferented and all the muscles, except two for recording, have been paralysed by nerve-section [35]. A single muscle isolatedly attached to the myograph, the rest of the musculature of both hind limbs having been paralysed and the isolated muscle itself deafferented, will still exhibit stepping, e.g. knee-extensor, in decerebrate preparation [35, 180].

(4) The automatic stepping of a hind limb under deep narcosis (cat) persists after cutting away the opposite half of the spinal cord in that limb region [37].

(5) The incidence of the turning-point, in short, the whole rhythm of the phase, both in the scratch and the stepping, is synchronous [168] throughout the entire field of musculature employed. The turning-point is not abrupt, either with the group or with the isolated deafferented muscle. Each phase presents a regular waxing and waning of activity.

(6) Unipolar faradization of the aboral face of the lateral column of the cut spinal cord, e.g. cervical region, will excite 'scratch' [148] or 'stepping' in the hind limbs [148], and does so in a deafferented hind limb [178]. As regards the stepping it can be bilateral under stimulation of one lateral column but is stronger in the ipselateral limb; it is of opposed phase in the two limbs, opening with flexion in the ipselateral limb, extension in the contralateral. Strengthening the spinal stimulation strengthens the movement and quickens the rhythm, accelerating the recurrence of the turning-points. Strychnine in subconvulsive dose greatly facilitates the scratch reflex. In the cross-area of the cervical cord the stepping spot lies in the dorsal depth of the lateral column. Concurrent stimulations of the two points right and left reinforce each other's effect on the hind limbs. The rhythm remains opposed in phase in the two limbs under the concurrent stimulation, unless the latter's strength is pushed, when the rhythm can become synchronously similar in phase, i.e. galloping [191].

(7) In the chronic spinal preparation (e.g. dog, cat) stepping of the spinal hind limbs sets in when they hang pendent, thus practically excluding exteroceptive stimulation. It is better obtained with the spine vertical than horizontal, i.e. better with the inguinal fold and hip more stretched. This stepping persists, e.g. 20 minutes at a time, but stops at once [178] if either limb be passively supported in slight flexion at knee and hip, e.g. by the observer's finger placed gently under the knee as the flexion phase at hip subsides, so that the limb no longer drops pendent. Both limbs then cease to step. This passive foreclosure of the extension phase in one limb annuls in some way the supervention of the active flexion phase of the other limb, and this

latter hangs inactive. The 'stepping' remains thus suspended indefinitely, until the passively supported limb is, by removal of the support, allowed to drop into passive extension at hip and knee; then active flexion at once occurs in the other limb, and the stepping of both limbs recommences. This reaction is clearly reflex and appears as a converse to the lengthening reaction of the decerebrate preparation, where passive flexion of the tonic knee provokes, along with reflex relaxation of its own extensor, reflex contraction of the contralateral knee- and ankle-extensors.

(8) The turning-point can be manufactured reflexly. This can be done by exerting on the motoneurones of the muscle the two opposed influences of reflex excitation and reflex inhibition concurrently and continuously and with a balanced intensity by stimulation of two symmetrical afferent nerves right and left, e.g. in the two hind limbs [36, 88, 180] (Fig. 63). Not only the turning-point but the regular succession of waxing and waning alternate phases of contraction and relaxation is thus producible. Proprioceptive reactions from the rhythmically contracting and relaxing muscle itself are not required for this. It is obtainable with the completely de-afferented muscle [180]. Though dependent on the two streams of centripetal impulses the effect is essentially central. With the paired knee-extensors right and left of the decerebrate preparation the rhythms right and left can be synchronized together, but the concurrent phases are opposite in direction. By adjusting the strength of stimulation right and left, the one extensor can be kept inhibitorily relaxed while the other is in quick rhythmic action, i.e. one leg is kept drawn up while the other runs [180].

(9) In the decerebrate preparation under rigidity the scratch reflex and stepping are less easily obtainable than in the spinal. This may be because the limb flexors are then commonly under inhibitory restraint [196], while conversely the limb-extensors are under excitatory reinforcement. But in the decerebrate preparation stepping can be evoked by concurrent faradization of paired afferent nerves, e.g. peroneals in the hind limbs right and left. In the spinal preparation stimulation of one hind foot provokes stepping of the crossed limb; but in decerebrate

rigidity maintained crossed extension usually replaces the crossed stepping of the spinal preparation.

(10) The scratch reflex and 'stepping' can be reflexly suppressed by evoking other reflexes in the limb, e.g. steady extension of the limb, or steady flexion can displace and exclude them. Stimulation of a point in the cut face of the cervical spinal cord can also arrest the stepping [191]—this point corresponds in the topography of the spinal cross-area with the region of the vestibulo-spinal tract. It arrests the stepping and evokes extension of the ipselateral hind limb.

The nervous mechanism answerable for the essential rhythmicity of the scratch reflex and stepping seems a central spinal one, not requiring *rhythmic* impulsion from outside. For spinal stepping Graham Brown [38] has especially insisted on this. That its rhythm can be regulated and influenced by secondary reflexes occasioned in the limb by phases of the act 'stepping' itself is indicated by observations, e.g. (7) above. Such influence has been traced to proprioceptive reflexes [178]. Co-operation of skin reflexes is certainly not essential for stepping. 'Spinal' stepping occurs readily and indeed best when the hind limbs are off the ground and without support. In the cat, normal except for desensitization of the feet, the stepping act is executed despite that desensitization with surprising approach to apparent normality. With all four feet desensitized the animal will walk the rungs of a horizontally placed 12-foot ladder quickly without stumble or hesitation and without a glance at its feet [178]. The bird after complete deafferentation of one foot will sleep standing perched on the deafferentated foot [47]. The contact of the sole with the ground, however, reinforces the extensors of the limb [63, 145]. The extensor thrust of the limb signifying the gallop [178] is excited by plantar pressure, or even from hairlets on the underside of the foot.

The stepping of the spinal hind limbs has been compared with the rhythmic activity of respiration [38, 178]. Graham Brown has shown that narcosis and asphyxia favour its occurrence, and that it may then arise autocthonously in the centre. The excitation is, however, commonly by stimulation either of peripheral afferents or of intraspinal descending paths which are, in relation to the spinal motor centre likewise afferent.

The production of the rhythmic reflex by continuous stimulation of the lateral column of the cut spinal cord may resemble the bilateral stimulation of symmetrical afferent nerves in so far that the descending spinal fibres stimulated include some of opposed effect, i.e. excitatory-inhibitory, on extensors and flexors respectively.

In all these rhythmic reflexes the incidence of the turning-point is synchronous throughout all the large field of musculature employed. In 'stepping' the turning-point is synchronous throughout the musculature of both hind limbs. This suggests as feature of the central mechanism an internuncial relay of wide distribution. There might be supposed for such a penultimate relay a slow depolarization wave on the analogy of the rhythmic potential waves discovered by Adrian and Buytendijk [12] in the brain stem of the teleost. It is noteworthy that the 'scratch' [176] and stepping [38] are facilitated by asphyxial conditions. The phasing of these alternating reflexes can be affected by the proprioceptive and other stimuli which they generate—as well as of course by many other extrinsic stimuli—but their phasing is not *caused* by peripheral stimuli [38]. The self-generated proprioceptive stimuli of the muscles which take part in progression can regulate the act but are not essential to its rhythm.

Another form taken by the transition from one reflex act to another is where a movement leads to and is succeeded by a posture. This item of reflex co-ordination is well exhibited in the decerebrate preparation where a crossed extensor reflex has as its sequel, following withdrawal of the stimulation of the crossed reflex itself, a persistence of the active knee-position reached although the stimulus provoking it has ceased. Here in the extensor muscle an autogenous proprioceptive postural reflex appends itself to the exteroceptively excited crossed reflex. The one merges into the other so smoothly and fully that there may be even in the plateau line of the myograph nothing to indicate where one ended and the other began. It is coalescence rather than a suffixing; it is as though the autogenous reflex of the muscle accompanied the exteroceptively evolved reflex contraction of the muscle and stood revealed only when the latter on withdrawal of the exteroceptive stimulus died out. It illustrates the aphorism that posture accompanies movement like its shadow. The myogram plateau, isometric or isotonic, may for a time remain unaltered though the postural reflex has replaced the exteroceptive which induced it. Reflex inhibition, however, detects a difference; the postural remainder is the more inhibitable.

Here the co-ordinative process operating the transition or liaison consists in attaching an autogenous proprioceptive reflex of the muscle itself (the shortening reaction) to the reflex, exteroceptive or other, which brings that muscle into action. It is noteworthy that for this the 'decerebrate', not the spinal, is the preparation of predilection, i.e. prespinal centres in support of spinal.

DECEREBRATE RIGIDITY

Recourse is taken to ablation of portions of the central nervous system the better to isolate for observation the functions of the reduced remainder. But the central organ is too intricate in spatial arrangement to allow of gross mutilation without distortion as well as simplification of its functions. Removal of the cerebral hemispheres above the thalami in cat and dog still allows, on recovery from the anaesthetic, assumption of the sitting or the standing posture. This it does in virtue of a system of reflexes, largely labyrinthine, the 'righting' reflexes (Magnus), which co-operate with a further set, postural and proprioceptive, in the wide sense of that term, executive of attitude. If the ablation be made further aboral, e.g. by transection between the anterior and posterior colliculi, there appears instead of the fairly normal posturing of the thalamus preparation a characteristic extensor rigidity, 'decerebrate rigidity'. The animal then, in absence of external stimulation, remains with extended limbs and neck, whether set on its side, or prone, or supine. If placed upright upon its feet it retains the erect position so given it. The weight of the various parts is then supported by the continuous contraction of muscles counteracting gravity. The limbs do not give way, the head is erect, the neck does not sink, the back does not yield, the tail does not drop, the lower jaw is kept lifted against the upper. All that system of musculature which posturally resists gravity in the erect position exhibits steady contraction. Its contraction is reflex [159], and proprioceptive reflexes play a great role in its production. For the fore-limb the proprioceptive reflexes are from the head mainly, the labyrinthine [141, 142]. For the hind limb the proprioceptive reflexes are from the extensor muscles themselves mainly, for with these, if in a sample muscle exhibiting the rigidity the afferent fibres be cut, the rigidity contraction disappears from that muscle, though affected little or not at all by the cutting of other afferents [170]. The reflex contraction in these extensors is therefore autogenous in source being traceable to proprioceptors of the reacting muscle itself, although it is reinforceable, and replaceable for short spells, by headward proprioceptive reflexes from the neck, &c. In the fore-limb, however, these latter altogether predominate.

The preparation does not possess in the same adequate measure, as does the thalamic, the power to assume or to adjust its erect posture. It has not the same righting reflexes. Laid on its side or inverted it cannot raise itself to the sitting or standing position.

Other differences between it and the thalamic preparation are: the marked pseud-affective condition of the latter, e.g. as reactions to skin stimuli, lashing of tail-tip, pilomotor erection in tail, 'aggressive' vocalization, unsheathing of claws, dilatation of pupil, retraction of lips, springing and running action of limbs. The threshold for skin stimuli does not seem regularly lower than in the intercollicular preparation, but each reaction to the supraliminal stimulus is followed in the thalamic preparation by a short train of muscular acts largely locomotor, and of pseud-affective character.

The posture maintained in decerebrate rigidity resembles 'standing' in that it presents a continuous (postural) contraction of the greater share of all that synergic system of muscles which by equipoising gravity in the erect position executes and maintains the standing attitude. The chief departure is in the apex of the limb, which is relatively limp. But normal standing is a geotropic reaction, and this reflex 'rigidity' is not *per se* a geotropic reaction. The rigidity persists when the animal is laid on its side and after excluding the specific geotropic receptors, the labyrinths [178]. Nevertheless in it the musculature for standing is operated reflexly and throughout practically all its manifold details and synergy, although the accessory righting reflexes are almost wanting.

With the preparation on its feet in the erect position a reflex posturally maintaining its attitude is the 'stretch reflex' [119, 187]. This is so to say potentially geotropic, because as limbs, neck, tail, or jaw yield or droop under gravity, each such yield stretches the corresponding antigravity muscles and these react by postural contraction to it; and these are the muscles which play the grand rôle normally in execution of the erect posture throughout the body. Its excitatory reactions may be so enhanced in decerebrate rigidity that the 'lengthening reaction' dependent on proprioceptively excited self-inhibition [173] of the limb-extensor may in some instances be no longer obtainable, proving ineffective against the high degree of tonic excitation. This ineffectiveness argues against the 'lengthening reaction' being a 'pain' reflex or the stimulus which provokes it being of 'painful' nature, i.e. in the sense of acting via nociceptive ('pain') afferents in the muscle. Usually the extensor tonus of decerebrate rigidity is moderate enough to allow readily of the 'lengthening reactions'. The degree of rigidity varies from experiment to experiment probably owing to small differences in the level or details of the trauma. With moderate rigidity the condition shows good static stretch reflexes of the extensors, and lowness of threshold and free after-discharge for the extensor reflexes generally, coupled with, for the flexor reflexes, a threshold much higher and a response less free than obtain for them in the 'spinal' state.

But not uncommonly the 'rigidity' is more extreme. The 'standing' of the decerebrate preparation is then an exaggeration and caricature of normal standing. Along with the strong tonus of the extensors the flexors, e.g. semitendinosus, sartorius, and tibialis anticus, instead of reacting to a pluck by the simple 'pluck reflex' [13] may respond with a short clonus. There is an admixture of flexor and extensor superactivity. As with general stimulation of a bared afferent nerve-trunk, so here an unnatural commingled functional activity results: so also here a particular functional component of the admixt functional condition is salient and dominates. That dominant here is the activity of the postural proprioceptive vestibular system which operates the antigravity muscles, broadly taken, the executive of 'standing'. The rigidity is therefore synergic and co-ordinate in many respects; it is also artificial and complex, and at times even swings over into predominance of flexor tonus [16]. Such flexor tonus is certainly at times the accompaniment of haemorrhage with clot accumulated in and over the fourth ventricle. Commonly, however, it presents broadly, and often with approach to purity, the neuromuscular system for standing—parted it is true from its geotropic receptor—and it presents that system in postural activity. The condition is not, however, fully tantamount to a simply, in the Jacksonian sense, released, pure, uncomplicated, and unmutilated exhibition of standing. Inferences drawn from its analysis can only be applied to normal standing with reserve.

THE SPINAL STATE

The spinal state obtaining after removal of the brain serves so commonly for study of reflexes, the question rises how far it and its reactions represent within their measure a normal co-ordination. Severance of the cord in higher mammals (cat, dog, monkey) produces at once a limp quietude of the skeletal muscles aboral from the transection; and even when the whole segmental length of the cord is so included. This muscular inactivity comprises absence of active attitude. The decapitated cat thus contrasts with the decapitated frog; the latter within a few minutes takes and maintains the squatting posture, less perfectly it is true in the fore-quarters than the hind. The 'spinal' cat contrasts perhaps even more with the cat 'decerebrated' by intercollicular transection of the brain stem. In this latter subsequent spinal transection has as its aboral consequence immediate disappearance of the extensor rigidity along with the lengthening and shortening reactions and Philippson's reflex, and a rise in threshold and fall in supraliminal response of the crossed extensor reflexes: conversely, an immediate and progressive fall in threshold with augmented volume of the direct flexion reflex [196]. The extensor excitation and facilitation which are thus removed aborally by the spinal transection are of prespinal origin because transection even half-way up the bulb is followed aborally by the same change. The extensor activity requires mainly the vestibular nucleus of the bulb, whence it descends by an uncrossed path, the vestibulo-spinal [99, 100, 170]. Headward of spinal severance in the decerebrate preparation there is some heightening of the reflex excitement of the extensors, e.g. the extensor rigidity of the fore-limbs is increased.

As to the marked facilitation [196] of the hind-limb flexor reflexes which in cat and dog follows spinal transection it is such that their threshold is lower than in either the intercollicular or the precollicular (thalamic) decerebrate preparation. The threshold continues falling for some hours after the severing of the cord, and the volume of the flexor contraction response as tested over a range of stimuli goes on increasing. This effect which holds for the cat and dog shows that in them the spinal condition, conversely from decerebrate rigidity, disturbs the extensor-flexor reflex-balance in favour of the flexors. It is therefore open to doubt whether the spinal preparation yields fair samples of co-ordination of a number of 'compounded' reflexes: thus its stepping is sometimes executed by the flexors alone without co-operation by the extensors [35].

Turning from cat and dog to a yet higher mammalian type, namely monkey, the paucity of spinal reflex action after severance of the spinal cord is striking [160]. It applies to the flexors as well as to the extensors. As for the latter even the knee-jerk, which in the spinal cat, although devoid of postural accompaniment and easily inhibitable, never defaults, is in the spinal monkey usually unelicitable for some hours or days following mid-thoracic transection; and its return is feeble and uncertain. Very occasionally, it is true, it does not completely disappear at all. The flexor reflexes, differently from their spinal condition in cat and dog, are here greatly depressed, sometimes even down to extinction [160]. Thus the reflex response of the ankle flexor to ipsilateral popliteal nerve as afferent which in the acute spinal cat will yield a contraction of 80 per cent. of the total muscle, in the acute spinal monkey sometimes yields no measurable contraction whatsoever. The spinal depression in the monkey therefore, besides being more severe, presents a qualitative difference from that of cat and dog.

The difference is rather widened than removed when regard is had to the course of events subsequent to transection. In cat and dog the reflex activity of the separated cord commonly improves for a period even of many weeks following the transection. Any such improvement if it occur in the monkey is much less. In the dog and cat the response to a spring clip on the foot is in the early period a simple flexion of the limb, and becomes later a reflex train of vigorous alternating flexion-extension and abduction-adduction which may not subside until it has freed the foot. Of the extensor muscles the 'quick' ones recover the less and the more slowly (p. 59). The crossed extension reflex becomes elicitable though not well maintained. The 'lengthening reaction' and Philippson's reflex become obtainable. In the ankle-extensor the static stretch reflex may be obtainable [67] though imperfect. In the dog the 'spinal' hind limbs if placed in the standing posture are found capable of maintaining the extended posture and supporting the weight of the hind quarters, even for minutes at a time. The 'spinal' standing is, however, subject to sudden lapses [178]. Vascular and visceral reflexes lie outside the scope of this book, yet we may note as to the improvement of reflex spinal activity gradually ensuing after high spinal severance that one of the most striking and measurable in the dog is recovery of the vasopressor reflexes operated from afferents behind the lesion, e.g. from a popliteal nerve. Hardly at first obtainable after cervical transection, they in the course of some weeks become elicitable and ample [168], and the general arterial pressure which had been dangerously lowered is in large measure restored.

This progressive improvement of spinal reflexes accruing during weeks, and even months, after spinal severance is commonly spoken of as 'subsidence of spinal shock'. The loss of function initially following a trauma of the central nervous system commonly is in part temporary; to explain its fugitive nature a factor often invoked is 'shock'. That in the nervous system a local traumatic lesion can irradiate disturbance some of which will be transient and subside is intelligible enough. Transient vascular derangement, local oedema, stages of inflammatory repair, will temporarily aggravate the results of a trauma. But that a trauma *per se* can continue for weeks and months as a focus radiating inhibitions to distant regions is a view with little now to recommend it. Trauma in the form of severance of a nerve-fibre is not a durable stimulus. Cut nerve-fibres in some cases cease to discharge impulses in a few seconds;

others of a certain kind persist for an hour or more (Adrian) [6].
From very early after completion of a trauma its effects upon
nervous function at a distance must depend solely on abeyance
of impulses normally current and, owing to paths broken and
sources annihilated, thenceforward lost. Impairment of local
function will then follow where impulses contributing (by summation) to motor excitation have been withdrawn, even though
they may have had in themselves but subliminal value: thus,
the impairment of hind-limb extensor reflexes after cutting off
vestibular influence by spinal transection. Conversely, the interruption of impulses contributory to inhibition can exalt reflex
activity: thus, the lower threshold and increased volume of
the flexor reflex aboral to spinal transection in decerebrate
rigidity.

The impairment of the extensor and vasopressor reflexes, so
marked an immediate sequel to cord section, shows that the
spinal centres for these after withdrawal of a main and more or
less continual stream of impulses normally incident on them
cannot for a time respond to the much reduced excitation hence-
forth available. Some gradual improvement does accrue during
the following weeks. After the break in their activity consequent
on the cord section the motoneurones may assume in course of
time a condition of lower threshold which renders them responsive to the reduced excitation available. Trophic changes
associated with function may enter here. There is, in neuro-
cytology, an analogy in the regressive chromatolytic changes in
motoneurones and Clarke-column cells induced by spinal severance, and in the course of weeks showing recovery [206].

In the laboratory the most extreme example of 'spinal shock'
is that presented by the monkey [101, 160]. There in the hind
limb not only extensor but flexor reflexes are scarcely obtainable; and lapse of time brings, so far as the skeletal muscles are
concerned, little recovery or acquisition of reflex reaction. The
neurocytological analogy might be to chromatolysis too severe
for repair. The skeletal muscles waste obviously. The condition by its greater severity suggests, more cogently than in cat
and dog and with more emphasis, that along with abeyance of
activity there supervenes a neuromuscular change amounting to
dystrophy. This, since consequent on functional isolation of the

spinal from the remaining nervous system, has been spoken of as 'isolation-dystrophy' [160, 209].

An interest attaches to this condition because of the monkey's closer likeness to man. The contrast between the effect of spinal transection on the hind-limb flexors in monkey and in cat and dog indicates a prespinal influence exerted in the higher animal upon the flexors which is wanting and relatively negligible in the lower. It is natural to correlate this with the more developed cortico-spinal tract of monkey.

The above suggests that, in order to shift control of a reflex effect from a spinal to a supraspinal mechanism, all that is needful is so to reinforce the supraspinal factor in the excitation of the 'motor centre' that the spinal factor (e.g. spinal afferents) sinks in its share of the summated total so as no longer of itself to supply enough excitation to operate the effect. It may be that the spinal afferents can still exert the effect indirectly by enlisting the developed supraspinal mechanism ('long-circuiting' [95]), but after loss of this latter they do not of themselves suffice. Summation and the manner of production of the reflex threshold being what they are, all that is anatomically required for the shift of control from one route to the other is an alteration in the relative density of the axone terminals. Such change of density could secure, for instance, that the threshold of the flexion reflex become subject entirely to a supraspinal mechanism.

One inference fairly obtainable from the reactions of the 'spinal condition' and bearing upon it as a field for study of reflex co-ordination is the following. Where a reflex centre is concerned muscular quiescence may mean (a) either quiescence of the reflex organ as regards the muscle or (b) activity within the reflex organ producing there inhibition as regards the muscle. The quiescence of the skeletal musculature in the spinal mammal proves on analysis to mean quiescence of the reflex organ; it seems nowhere to predicate active inhibition. The study of co-ordination in the 'spinal' preparation has therefore a clean background of passive quiescence against which excitation can be shown uncomplicated and unhindered by residual inhibitory opposition to excitation.

This inference strengthens another. From lower animal types varied and energetic reflexes are obtainable in the 'spinal' condition. Thus, there are limb flexion and limb extension in the frog, some limb extension but mainly limb flexion in cat and dog. On turning to types closer to man, e.g. monkey, it may be that the marked default of such reflexes in these latter is due to untoward accessory conditions such as shock, inhibition, toxins, &c., rather than to fundamental disability of the spinal machinery for such reactions. Yet, facing the facts, there seems no valid evidence that purely spinal reflexes like those demonstrable in the spinal cat and dog are present in the monkey. There is no evidence of residual inhibition at work in its spinal state, and the reflexes obtainable in cat and dog cannot be elicited. They are not there. It seems clear that in the higher animal type supraspinal factors of co-ordination have taken over the province of what in lower types mainly belonged to the spinal executive. In the higher type the spinal executive when unsupported no longer exercises the offices which in the lower type it does. In so far as concerns the skeletal musculature there is between the 'spinal condition' of the dog on the one hand and of the monkey on the other a difference hardly less, although converse in direction, than that obtaining between them in respect of cerebral development.

The higher the mammalian type the less of purely reflex function will there be which a spinal transection can release. Whether anything complete, in the sense of being an act executed as regards its co-ordination not less successfully in the spinal than in the normal intact animal, is still retained at spinal level in the higher mammal is doubtful. In the frog it may be that there is. In the cat some of the pinna reflexes examined in this respect reveal to inspection little difference in their execution in the bulbo-spinal and in the intact cat respectively [183]. This suggests that in the intact cat their bulbo-spinal machinery suffices and runs for itself, and that higher centres release or prevent but do not interfere in detail. The point of view reached in this respect amounts to that which has long been held for the respiratory act of lung-ventilation. The pinna reflex executes a very simple act for a very simple effect; but it is doubtful whether in the higher animal type, e.g. monkey, even so simple an act remains purely bulbo-spinal.

CONCLUDING REMARKS

We may ask in conclusion whether from the attempted analysis of the simpler reflexes anything like a general principle emerges fundamental to co-ordination. In some degree there does. That important and practically omnipresent factor in co-ordination, namely adjustment of quantity of contraction, presents itself (and the more so as the scale of reflex complexity is ascended) as the resultant commonly of two interacting antagonistic central processes, excitation and inhibition (cf. Figs. 53, 62). The degree of activity of a motoneurone corresponds with the algebraical sum of the opposed influences of excitation and inhibition convergent upon it.

It is true that for physiological experiment the nervous system, purposely curtailed in extent, even to retention of perhaps but one afferent channel, and that one active only while artificially stimulated, exhibits reflex excitation freed in many cases from concurrent inhibition. It is true also that that central excitation can be graded, by grading the stimulus, and that so also can inhibition. But under intact natural conditions we have to think of each motoneurone as a convergence-point about which summate not only excitatory processes fed by converging impulses of varied provenance arriving by various routes, but also inhibitory influences of varied provenance and path; and that there at that convergence-place these two opposed influences finally interact.

The two convergent systems themselves, one excitatory, one inhibitory, make of the entrance to the final common path, which we may accept the motoneurone as constituting, a collision-field for joint algebraically summed effect. In the higher vertebrate rarely is either member of this paired system, excitatory-inhibitory, wholly quiet when its fellow is active, for their relation to stimuli is reciprocal. The opposition between the effects of the two on the motoneurone is quantitative, and the grade of functional activity or inactivity of the motoneurone reflects this quantitative interaction. Whether the excitatory has the upper hand, or whether the inhibitory, commonly both are at work, and the functional state of the motoneurone indexes the net result from the two.

This statement can find justification and illustration in such a simple instance as that of the extensor muscles. With them we know that the mechanical action of the muscle itself affects reflexly the activity of its own motoneurones. The muscle's contraction by pulling on its own tendon can and does produce reflex excitation of itself (*autogenous excitation*), indeed this appears as one basis of its reflex tone. Active contraction of the muscle can also stimulate certain receptors in it which develop reflex inhibitory restraint (*autogenous inhibition*) of its own motoneurones. The ataxy of *tabes dorsalis* with its impairment of tone and its unchecked muscular momentum (Fig. 64) illustrates well how constantly each natural act rests for its normal execution on a collaboration between concurrent excitation and inhibition.

The picture of an excitatory system convergent upon the motoneurone and gathering impulses from manifold sources and paths, varying in extent and power with the set or sets of receptors in action and with the series of centres involved, offers no difficulty and the text-books furnish for it abundant diagrams. In respect, however, to the inhibitory system which the principle of action now before us requires us to envisage as more or less a counterpart and counterpoise to the excitatory against which it acts, a certain ambiguity enters the picture. Central inhibition is by experiment clearly shown to have a locus closely circumjacent to the motoneurone itself, i.e. in terms of reflex direction immediately upstream from that. There the convergent inhibitory system will certainly act. But as to whether on its way thither the inhibitory system also at other links in its neurone chain, for instance further upstream and headward (for some of its chains are long), develops inhibition which can influence the motoneurone remains still obscure. Except at the locus of the motoneurone central inhibition is little known to actual experiment, apart from somewhat indirect evidence for the bulbar vasomotor and respiratory centres.

Fundamental in the co-ordinative regulation of the motoneurone is the combined action on it of the summed excitations of the moment pitted against the concurrent summed inhibitions. Each individual motoneurone is individually dealt with thus. Hence these two opposed and separately gradable influences which by antagonistic interaction also mutually grade together, make the motoneurone and therefore the motor unit their unit of operation. The foundation of the quantitative grading is based on the individual motor unit. The musculature as a whole being composed additively of motor units the co-ordinative taxis takes expression in the musculature as a whole as an additive effect.

The range of excitation and inhibition experimentally observable in the individual motoneurone is more extensive than the mechanical response of the muscle-fibres can follow. The rate of firing of the motoneurone under summed excitation can exceed the rate which produces full tetanic tension of the motor unit. Heights of excitation therefore occur in the nervous centres greater than the skeletal muscle-fibre can commensurately express [191]. If this seems wasteful of central activity we may remember that additional excitation exerted on a motoneurone whose muscle-fibres are already driven maximally for tetanic contraction is not necessarily wasted. That surplus remains still a contribution to co-ordination because further excitation offers a further resistance to inhibition. Conversely, an added inhibition in the case of an already quiescent neurone although in one sense wasted, is a further protection which co-ordination may need against excitation. In times of crisis the dilemma lies between strong actions and the very strength of the action taken may serve to safeguard it against interruption.

APPENDIX I
STRUCTURAL FEATURES OF MUSCLE RECEPTORS IN MAMMALS

FROM one-third to one-half of the fibres composing any nerve (other than a branch of a cranial nerve) distributed entirely to skeletal muscle are processes of cells situated in dorsal root ganglia, as can be proved by degeneration experiments [158] (Fig. 67).[1] These fibres are therefore afferent, and they carry impulses to the central nervous system from proprioceptive endings in muscles and tendons and from other deep structures. They terminate peripherally in various ways and have a number of important functions. They inform consciousness of the position and the movements of the different parts of the body; they subserve reflexes like the knee-jerk in response to passive stretch; there is good evidence that some of them are stimulated by active contraction; endings in the muscles and joints of the neck and trunk initiate attitudinal and righting reflexes affecting almost the whole body; and in some circumstances (e.g. cramp) pain may be evoked from muscles and tendons.

Of the organs in which these afferent fibres are distributed, the most complex and interesting are the *muscle-spindles* (Fig. 68). The mammalian muscle-spindle [107, 149, 158] measures from 0·75 mm. to 4 mm. in length and is from 80μ to 200μ in diameter at its widest part. Its long axis lies parallel to the muscle-fibres in which it is embedded. Situated as a rule in the fleshy parts of the muscles, spindles are plentiful in the limb-muscles, where their number has been estimated to be sufficient to account for almost two-thirds of all the afferent nerve-fibres of those muscles. They appear to be absent (at all events in this particular form) from the facial muscles and from the intrinsic muscles of the tongue and larynx, and, in many animals, from the external ocular muscles.

Each spindle consists of a bundle of from two to twelve intra-fusal muscle-fibres enclosed within a capsule of circularly arranged fibrous tissue. A distinct space, which may be 40μ to 60μ wide in the equatorial region, separates the capsule from its contents. This space contains lymph, and is bridged across

[1] See plate facing p. 99.

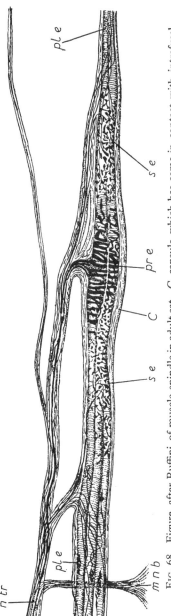

Fig. 68. Figure, after Ruffini, of muscle-spindle in adult cat. *C*, capsule, which has come in contact with intrafusal muscle-fibres owing to dehydration of periaxial lymph-space by glycerine used in teasing preparation; *n.tr*, nerve trunk; *mn.b*, motor-nerve bundle, ending exclusively in motor-end plates *pl.e*, in muscle-fibres; *pr.e*, primary ending of afferent fibre; *s.e*, secondary endings.

by delicate septa which unite the capsule with the axial sheath of connective tissue investing the bundle of muscle-fibres (Fig. 69).

Two or three rather small muscle-fibres enter the spindle at its proximal end. Within the spindle they tend to split lengthwise, each producing perhaps three daughter fibres which become tendinous as they approach the distal pole of the organ. The structure of the intrafusal fibres differs from that of ordinary muscle-fibres. For a considerable part of their length they are circular in cross-section, with a diameter of $6\,\mu$ to $28\,\mu$; their nuclei are often embedded in their thickness; commonly it is only the marginal sheet of their substance which is striated; and the striations are coarser than in the neighbouring ordinary fibres. In the equatorial region of the spindle the striation is obscured by a large collection of nuclei. The afferent nerve endings are found in this region and differ from motor endplates in never being hypolemmal.

The nerve-supply of muscle-spindles is derived from two sources. The intrafusal fibres possess motor end-plates supplied by small unbranched medullated nerve-fibres, which degenerate on section of ventral spinal roots (Onanoff; Cipollone). After severance of the nerve to a muscle, the muscle-fibres in the spindles do not atrophy, as do ordinary muscle-fibres. Each spindle also receives, on the average, three to four large medullated fibres, even up to $18\,\mu$ in diameter, which degeneration experiments have shown to be dorsal root ganglion fibres [158]. These pierce the capsule from the side, usually between the equator and the proximal pole, and do not lose their myelin sheaths until they have crossed the periaxial space and reached the intrafusal muscle-fibres. They branch freely at nodes of Ranvier, and their terminal filaments, which may be connected with several intrafusal muscle-fibres, are larger in diameter than the parent nerve-fibre.

The axis-cylinders of the afferent fibres end in one of two ways in connexion with the intrafusal muscle-fibres. The largest of them, after losing their myelin sheaths just before actually meeting a muscle-fibre, become flat and broad like ribbons. The ribbon either divides into two and wraps itself round the intrafusal fibre as a spiral, in which case the turns lie

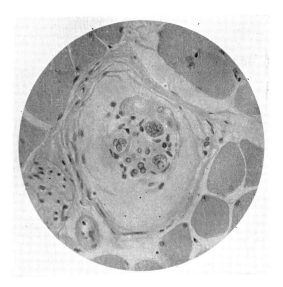

Fig. 69 A. Transverse section of muscle-spindle in equatorial region, showing fibrous capsule, lymphatic space bridged by septa, and intrafusal muscle-fibres. Outside the capsule is ordinary muscle-tissue.

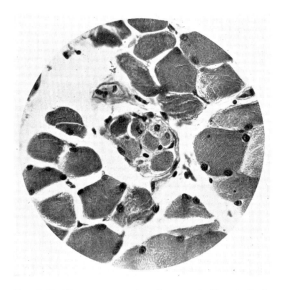

Fig. 69 B. Transverse section of same spindle as in 69 A, near one pole. The lymphatic space is hardly visible.

very close together at the middle of the ending and gradually open out to terminate in free ends, or it runs lengthwise along the surface of the muscle-fibre giving off a succession of ribbon-like rings which encircle the fibre. Together these constitute Ruffini's annulo-spiral endings. The smaller afferent fibres are both myelinate and amyelinate. The myelinate enter the spindle at some distance from the entrance of those that have already been described, and divide into secondary branches which, like the latter, are distributed to the muscle-fibres near the equator of the spindle. Their naked axis-cylinders ramify around and upon the intrafusal muscle-fibres to form the elaborate and delicate structures which are suggested by the name 'flower-spray ending' (Ruffini). It is usual to find both these types of ending close together on the same intrafusal fibre. The non-medullated fibres accompany the primary sensory bundle of the spindle and reach the intrafusal muscle-fibres by crossing the periaxial lymph-space of the spindle. Their most usual ending is as minute rings or plates epilemmally placed among the nuclei of the *sheath* of the intrafusal muscle-fibre, often in the region of the annulo-spiral ending of Ruffini.

In the majority of mammalian muscles the muscle-spindle is the ending by which afferent nerve-fibres enter most closely into relation with muscle-fibres. It is probable that the adequate stimulus is active contraction or passive stretch or both.

Weiss and Dutil [207] have described branches of a single nerve-fibre in the cat being distributed, one to a muscle-spindle, and another to a Golgi tendon-organ.

Rather similar, though much simpler, spindle-organs in the frog respond to passive stretch [131, 132]. That there are receptors responsive to active contraction has been proved in a number of ways [53, 55, 62].

Muscle-spindles have not been found in the *eye-muscles* of the cat, the monkey, and many other species. These muscles are, however, plentifully supplied with endings of afferent type [70, 201] which are derived, as degeneration experiments have proved, from fibres of the third, fourth, and sixth cranial nerves. The receptors are found in intimate relation with the contractile muscle-fibres, as well as in tendon and connective tissue. To the former group belong fine arborizations on the surface of the muscle-fibres, and peculiar endings at the junction of muscle and

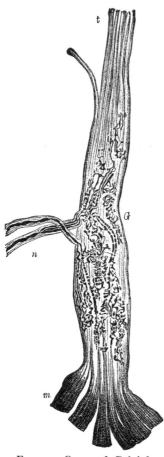

tendon. These are the terminal filaments of branching medullated fibres and they ramify for a short distance along the surface of the muscle-fibres, which they approach by recurving from the direction of the tendon. The ramifications tend to lie approximately parallel to the long axis of the muscle-fibre.

In the tendons of mammalian muscles the most characteristic receptors are the tendon-spindles or *Golgi organs* (Fig. 70). These are found in all tendons close to their muscular origin. They appear to be specially frequent in tendon bundles arising from muscle-spindles. Each organ (see [109]) consists of a number of tendon fasciculi surrounded by a lymph space and enclosed in a fusiform or cylindrical fibrous capsule. It is supplied by one or two myelinate nerve-fibres, which are smaller than those of muscle-spindles and than most of the motor fibres from ventral roots. After entering the capsule the fibres break up into smaller branches and ultimately lose their myelin sheaths. They terminate in a rich arborization in the tendon bundle. The whole structure may exceed 0·5

FIG. 70. Organ of Golgi from human Tendo Achillis. Gold chloride preparation (Ciaccio). *m*, muscle-fibres; *t*, tendon-bundles; *G*, Golgi's organ; *n*, two nerve-fibres passing to it.

mm. in length. As tendon is not contractile and is almost inextensible, there can be little doubt but that the adequate stimulus for these organs is mechanical tension on the tendon in which they lie. They are probably excited both by passive and by active tension.

Pacinian corpuscles, supplied by medullated nerve-fibres, are of frequent occurrence in the neighbourhood of tendinous insertions. They are also found in the fascia covering muscles, and sometimes embedded in the fleshy tissue of the muscles themselves. Pressure undoubtedly constitutes their adequate stimulus [11]. A rather simpler and less frequent type of encapsulated ending, which probably also responds to mechanical stimuli, is the *Golgi-Mazzoni corpuscle*. This is met with in tendons and in the sheaths both of tendons and of muscles. In addition, comparatively undifferentiated *free nerve-endings* occur in the connective tissue of muscles. These perhaps subserve pain, and may be the endings of some of the amyelinate afferent fibres which Nevin [133] finds present in nerves distributed to muscle.

In the existing state of knowledge it would evidently be rash to attempt to specify the reflex functions of any of the proprioceptive endings which have been described. Nor is it known which among them subserve 'muscle-sense'.

FIG. 71. Schema of end-organs in mammalian muscle (Denny-Brown). The original figure has been modified to include fusimotor fibres. Each muscle-fibre contributes a slip of tendon to the aponeuroses of origin and insertion. In muscles such as tenuissimus, many muscle-fibres are joined end to end and innervated by one motor nerve fibre. Finely medullated afferent nerve fibres (1) have free endings in the connective tissue, chiefly near blood vessels, to which they are distributed with the non-medullated sympathetic plexus (2). Four motor nerve fibres (3, 3, 3, 3) are drawn as innervating 23 muscle-fibres so that each fibre receives only one motor end-plate. Many more muscle-fibres are innervated from each motoneurone (Ref. 38) than can be shown here, and the muscle-fibres innervated by each motoneurone are scattered. The schematic muscle-spindle has three slender muscle-fibres, two of which receive motor terminations (MT) from independent small (fusimotor) motor fibres (4, 4), and one from an ultraterminal branch from an end-plate of an extra-fusal muscle-fibre.

Approximately one third of the nerve fibres in the 'motor' nerve (MN) are afferent fibres. An annulo-spiral (primary) ending of a large afferent fibre (5) encircles the central region (AS) of the muscle-fibres in the equator of the muscle-spindle. Many spindles also receive one or more branched 'flower-spray' (secondary) endings (FS) innervated by a smaller afferent fibre (6). No attempt is made here to portray more simple spindle muscle-fibres with a secondary instead of a primary zone and with more simple trailing types of motor end-plate. The Golgi tendon-organ (TO) receives the insertion of a small number of muscle-fibres which are innervated by different motor units, thus arranged to sample their tension development. Its afferent fibre (7) is large, but on the average slightly smaller than that of the annulo-spiral ending (cf. Fig. 73). The organ has a delicate ensheathing capsule. Both spindle and tendon-organ receive the termination of one or two sympathetic fibres in their equatorial regions.

Soleus muscle in the cat has an average of 56 muscle-spindles and 31 tendon-organs, medial gastroenemius, 70 spindles and 44 tendon-organs, and tibialis anticus a comparable number of each (Barker, Eldred et al., and Chin et al., in Muscle Receptors, ed. David Barker, Hong Kong, University Press, 1962). In addition each muscle has a few (5–7) scattered paciniform afferent endings near aponeuroses.

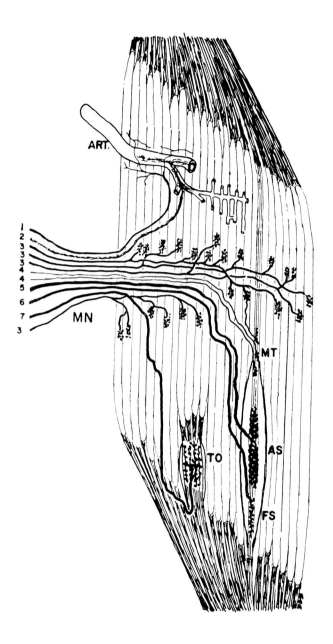

APPENDIX II

TABLE showing some common types of reflex reaction given by preparations (dog and cat) according to the level of section of the central neuraxis.

	Flexor muscles.	Extensor muscles.
Low spinal section: i.e. transection at or about level of last rib. i. 'acute spinal', i.e. some minutes or hours after transection.	Flexor reflex easily evoked. Tendon-jerk present ('pluck reflex'). Crossed inhibition.	Tendon-jerk present.
ii. 'Chronic spinal', i.e. some days, weeks, or months after transection.	Flexor reflex easily evoked. Tendon-jerk present. Crossed inhibition.	Tendon-jerk present. Imperfect stretch reflex (postural). Extensor thrust. Crossed extensor reflex.
Decerebrate: i.e. transection between anterior and posterior colliculi some minutes or hours previously.	Flexor reflex less readily evoked, but once evoked has considerable after-discharge. Tendon-jerk. Crossed inhibition.	Tendon-jerk with marked tonic after-discharge. Stretch reflex exaggerated and chief factor in decerebrate rigidity. Crossed extensor reflex easily obtained with long tonic after-discharge.

ANNOTATIONS TO THE
1972 REPRINT

I. THE REFLEX ARC

Note 1 (p. 3, line 11)

Nerve conduction velocity is now known to range from 0·72 (221) to approximately 120 metres per second. In this context discussion of nerve fibre nomenclature is in order. In the early studies by Gasser and Erlanger (217) with the aid of the oscilloscope three main groupings labelled A, B, and C were found. The A and B fibres were myelinated, the C fibres unmyelinated. Subsequently A fibres were subdivided into subgroups alpha, beta, gamma, and delta on the basis of recorded elevations in the compound action potential of a cutaneous nerve. In 1960 Gasser (223) finally clarified the content of a cutaneous nerve, specifically the saphenous nerve. The beta and gamma deflexions were shown to be artefacts due to the method of leading. Only the alpha and delta deflexions remained.

One difficulty was that there were in muscle nerves afferent fibres of higher conduction velocity than those called 'alpha' in cutaneous nerves. When some of the problems concerning reflex action of afferent fibres had been sorted out a new nomenclature was required. This need led to the coining of the designations Group I, Group II, and Group III. Alpha and delta fibres are comparable in diameter and conduction velocity to Group II and Group III afferent fibres in muscle nerves (Fig. 72). Group I fibres are unique to muscle nerves. They are divisible into Group IA fibres afferent from muscle spindles and Group IB fibres afferent from Golgi tendon organs. Group II afferent fibres also arise from the (secondary) receptors of muscle spindles (Fig. 73).

For some purposes and by some workers, alpha and delta fibres of cutaneous nerves are referred to as Group II and Group III fibres respectively. This practice is satisfactory certainly with respect to reflex physiology.

B fibres are present in the somatic nerves of the frog but not in those of the cat. They are of no further concern other than to note that they are among the preganglionic fibres of the autonomic nervous system.

There are in cutaneous nerves a high percentage of C fibres, but in muscle nerves their numbers are much fewer. Little is known of their action with respect to reflexes for which reason they receive little more than cursory consideration in these notes.

Motor fibre constitution of muscle nerves was established by Eccles and Sherrington (78). There are two groupings, of large and of small diameter, originally thought to pertain to large and small motor units

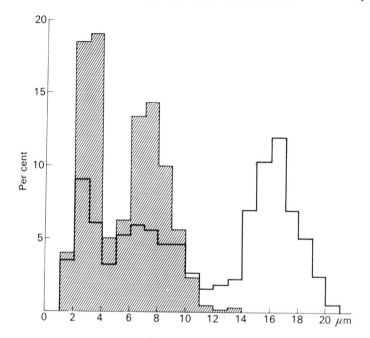

Fig. 72. Distribution of afferent fibres with respect to diameter in 'demotored' muscle nerves (heavy line). Motor fibres had been eliminated by virtue of degeneration subsequent to severance of ventral roots. The finer line and hatched area describes the distribution with respect to diametre of fibres in a cutaneous nerve. The three peaks of distribution are (from right to left) referred to as Groups I, II, and III respectively. Group I is confined to afferent fibres in muscle nerves.

respectively. The small fibres are now known to supply intrafusal muscle fibres of the muscle spindles (Leksell). Function of the groups now having been established the preferred names for the large and small fibres would be myomotor and fusimotor. There is evidence for two sub-groups within the fusimotor group. The term 'gamma efferents' must be recognized as referring to fusimotor fibres, but on several grounds is unhelpful. A newer development proposed at the Nobel Symposium of 1965 (212, 225) is to refer to motor fibres as alpha (myomotor), beta, and gamma (fusimotor), while reserving the terms Group I, Group II, and Group III (cutaneous and muscular) for afferent fibres. As alpha, beta, gamma (and delta) were designations of fibre groupings in cutaneous afferent fibres a new source of confusion in terminology may have arisen. The terms employed by P. B. C. Matthews (253) for the two groups of fusimotor fibres, namely

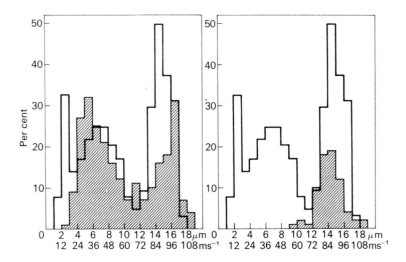

FIG. 73. At the left, distribution with respect to conduction velocity and hence to diametre of afferent fibres from A-type receptors (hatched area) as determined by Hunt superimposed upon the plot of distribution of afferent fibres in soleus nerve as determined histologically by Lloyd and Chang. There are two groups of A-type receptors (the primary and secondary spindle endings) connected to Group I and Group II afferent fibres. Note that the A-type fibres are in numbers biased toward the higher velocity, greater diametre, lower threshold members of the group. Group III fibres are not represented. At the right is the distribution found by Hunt of B-type receptors (hatched area) similarly displayed on the histological afferent fibre distribution in soleus nerve. B-type fibres are essentially confined to the Group I fibre band but are in distribution biased toward the lower velocity, lesser diametre, higher threshold members of the group. Groups II and III are not involved.

dynamic and static, are preferable. Thus it is suggested that myomotor, dynamic, and static fusimotor fibres constitute the most suitable terminology for motor fibres of the somatic system.

Note 2 (p. 3, line 35)

Although propagation *per se* is a matter of nerve-impulses, the influence of electrical current fields generated in one nucleus acting upon another nucleus or upon other cells within the same nucleus has been considered as being possibly an aspect of central control (12). The notion reappears from time to time (238, 259) and may have physiological significance. Opinions differ.

Note 3 (p. 4, line 10)

The Greek designation sigma (σ) has been universally replaced by the term millisecond, abbreviated as ms.

Note 4 (p. 5, line 3)

'Local excitatory state' is controversial. Some hold (e.g. 261) that at near threshold stimulation nerve produces an added response *sui generis* that can lead to discharge of an impulse. Others would regard the change as an abortive impulse and that the nerve in fact reacts to counter any change imposed upon it (251). It is now known that normal nerve displays a negative afterpotential and two positive afterpotentials, P_1 and P_2 in the nomenclature of Gasser (220). In brief, P_1 is the nerve reaction to the 'impulse' or spike potential. It is relatively immutable. P_2 is the nerve reaction to the negative afterpotential and, like it, is highly labile in its behaviour in varied circumstances. Lorente de Nó (251) has envisaged the nerve membrane as possessing two fractions: Q for quick and related to production of the spike potential (impulse) and P_1 reaction, and L for labile, related to negative afterpotential and P_2 reaction. This concept is extremely useful in consideration of elementary reflex transmission (238, 245–7) as well as for thinking concerning nerve itself (251). Importance came into being with respect to the spinal cord initially with the studies of Gasser and Graham (224) and of Hughes and Gasser (227, 228) and later with the discovery of excitatory and inhibitory postsynaptic potentials (cf. 214).

Note 5 (p. 5, line 11)

Although there is no evidence that the actual nature of nerve-impulses change, this could be so for one reason or another, such as functional block, decremental conduction, and changes in the relative values of the Q-fraction and L-fraction of membrane potential based upon the fact that electrotonic spread of the former is greatly confined in space by comparison with the latter. There is considerable information concerning precipitate decreases in conduction velocity where branching takes place (cf. 249). In reflex collaterals velocity of conduction is but a small and decrementing fraction of that in the parent primary afferent fibre. Such measurements of conduction time in afferent collaterals as have been made necessarily represent average conduction time from the parent fibre to an ill-defined point among the collaterals or, antidromically, from some ill-defined point in the collaterals to the parent afferent fibres. Added to these difficulties is controversy concerning the recordable potential changes that represent action at the primary afferent endings (214, 239, 247). Terminal velocity *sensu stricto* is of course zero.

Note 6 (p. 8, line 7)

Although the phrase '70 per sec' is perfectly clear the new terminology would refer to this as 70Hz. One hertz equals one cycle per second.

II. THE SPINAL GREY MATTER

Note 7 (p. 9, line 30)

It is virtually certain that the afferent impulses conduct directly from the peripheral to the central portions of the afferent neurones. Nevertheless there is strong evidence that they also enter the cell bodies in the dorsal root ganglia (264), perhaps in a manner comparable to that in which impulses at certain invertebrate axo-axonic synapses spread backward into the cell body of the postsynaptic unit. The most interesting recent study of afferent fibres comparing those on the distal and proximal sides of the dorsal root ganglion is that of Gasser (221) which, however, concerns C fibres. There are, in this case at any rate, differences.

Note 8 (p. 10, line 27)

In the second and third sacral segments of the spinal cord and possibly elsewhere there is now no question but that primary afferent fibres do indeed cross the medial longitudinal plane of the spinal cord (215, 216, 236, 247, 250). They establish direct connexions with motoneurones of the contralateral side and are inhibitory in their action upon those motoneurones. This statement, correct as it may be, is not unchallenged. Therefore the question of their exact site of ending might be considered debatable. It is certainly controversial.

Note 9 (p. 11, line 18)

In recent years the recurrent collateral or 'side fibre' has received great attention. It is said to form synaptic connexion with interneurones that have been designated 'Renshaw cells' by Eccles (214), after their discoverer. Renshaw cells in turn are supposed to act upon motoneurones. The usual method for investigating their action is by the use of antidromic volleys instigated by ventral root stimulation, although their response to orthodromic reflex stimulation has been seen. It is an interesting fact that excitability changes in inactive motoneurones located close to those activated by an antidromic impulse volley exactly match the current flows about the antidromically activated motoneurones (238). This would indicate that the current flows in the volume conductor about the active motoneurones might be responsible for the effects produced. Renshaw himself (259) considered the two possibilities, namely current flows and synaptic action, leaving the question open although expressing a preference for the current flow option. Synaptic action today is the more popular hypothesis.

A small ventral root discharge has been observed following an antidromic stimulation (233, 259). It is confined to the motoneurones that have been occupied by the antidromic volley and apparently is due to the fact that the motoneurone somata at the instant of inception are drawing current from their intramedullary axons which are simultaneously depolarized by virtue of their immense negative afterpotential. In any event the significance of this 'pseudoreflex' volley is related to events that occur after massive antidromic invasion. It is almost certainly of no account in reflex physiology.

Note 10 (p. 11, line 23)

A Golgi Type II cell is one in which the axone does not extend beyond the spread of the dendrites. Imprecise use of the term in recent years has not been helpful in the understanding of reflex mechanism. There are few if any Golgi Type II cells in the spinal cord although they are plentiful elsewhere. A reservation should probably be made with respect to the substantia gelatinosa Rolandi, of which relatively little is known.

Note 11 (p. 12, line 12)

Disintegration of Nissl substance or chromatolysis following severance of a neurone's axone is now recognized to be an aspect of regeneration rather than of degeneration (211).

Note 12 (p. 15, line 37)

Although controversy exists today this sentence and that ensuant are prescient with respect to reflex transmission. Central reflex time, as stated elsewhere, is the sum of central conduction time and synaptic delay. Its measurements show average central conduction time to be longer than was supposed (215, 217), therefore the duration of synaptic delay necessarily decreases. Some cling to the value for synaptic delay as being 0·5–1·0 ms. Others, considering measurements of average conduction velocity in the reflex collaterals, regard synaptic delay as possibly approaching zero (236, 247). As conduction in the fine reflex collaterals might continue beyond the point at which effective transmission takes place, the sum of conduction time and synaptic delay could, from a formal point of view and within the framework of definition, result in synaptic delay having a negative value.

III. THE FLEXOR REFLEX

Inasmuch as the flexor reflex was considered the archetype of the 'simple reflex', it naturally was employed to explore the elementary properties of the reflex arc (79–83). Subsequently flexor reflexes were found to contain in their minimum pathway at least one internuncial relay (234). Meanwhile the monosynaptic (or two-neurone) reflex had been established conclusively. The afferent fibres having direct access to the motoneurones, this reflex replaced the flexor reflex as the means for study of simple reflex action. The monosynaptic reflex arises in the Group IA afferent fibres of a given muscle, flexor or extensor, and by direct connexion to motoneurones reflects back to that same muscle. It is a fractional form of the stretch reflex (119). Fig. 74 illustrates the difference in character between a monosynaptic reflex (A) and a polysynaptic (flexor) reflex (B) as recorded in a ventral root subsequent to stimulation of a muscle nerve and of a cutaneous nerve respectively. As the stimuli were maximal for the myelinated afferent fibres there is added to the monosynaptic reflex in A a small polysynaptic reflex discharge.

With the advent of direct electrical recording of nerve impulses it became possible to discover how Eccles and Sherrington came to the conclusion that the flexor reflex contained a minimum direct pathway supplemented by parallel pathways of increasing numbers of serially positioned interneurones discharging in sequence to create at the motoneurone an incrementing state that was for convenience called *c.e.s.* There were no direct measurements of afferent conduction velocity. Thus they stimulated a peripheral nerve, noting the latency of muscle contraction. Then they stimulated a dorsal root, again noting the latency of muscle contraction. The difference in latency was taken to

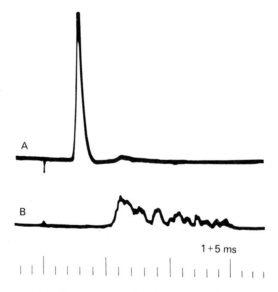

A

B

1 + 5 ms

FIG. 74. Reflex discharges recorded from a ventral root. A, response to maximal afferent stimulation of a muscle nerve. There is evident a prominent monosynaptic reflex followed by a small polysynaptic reflex. B, response similarly recorded to a maximal stimulation of a cutaneous nerve. There is in the latter no monosynaptic reflex but there is a prominent polysynaptic reflex discharge (flexor reflex).

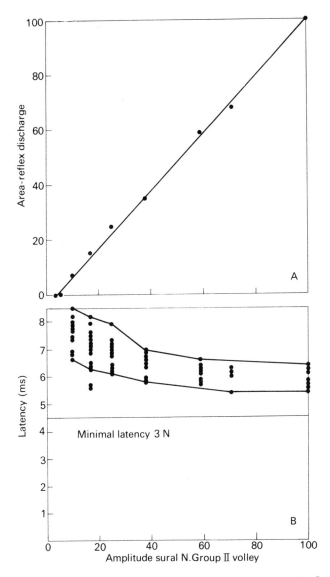

FIG. 75. Input–output relation in a Group II flexor reflex (A). Input–latency relationship in a number of trials (B). In curve A it is seen that the relation is linear once threshold at the motoneurones has been reached. Minimal latency as drawn in B at 4·5 ms represents the calculated reflex time for a pathway containing a single in-series internuncial relay. Clearly the flexor reflex experimentally is ineffective in its theoretical minimal pathway even in the circumstance of powerful synchronous afferent electrical stimulation. One may suppose that in natural circumstances an influence could be exerted through the minimal pathway upon whatever action was under way at the time.

be a measure of conduction time and hence of velocity. By stimulating the peripheral nerve they had indeed evoked a flexor reflex but on moving the stimulating electrodes to the dorsal root they had broken into the muscles own monosynaptic reflex pathway. The result was that the calculated afferent conduction time was too long and the central reflex time too short. It is of particular interest that a footnote (79, p. 515) stated that the afferent conduction time so measured would be valid only if the two reflexes were the same, which they proved not to be. Although direct measurements have clarified the situation it must be noted that the actual measurements by Eccles and Sherrington were as precise as could be made today.

Consideration of the chapter deals with two questions, that of the flexor reflex proper and that of the excitatory state at the motoneurone —questions that clearly must be separated.

Fig. 75 illustrates some of the characteristics of a Group II flexor reflex. Contained therein are (A) the manner of growth in size of the reflex discharge and (B) change in latency as an afferent volley (sural nerve) is increased from zero to maximum. The Group III flexor reflex is not represented, nor is that which is known to result from stimulation of C fibres. The upper plot (A) defines what is now known as the input–output relation. Once threshold is reached the relation for a Group II flexor reflex is linear (237, 254). The relation for a monosynaptic reflex is different.

Difference in input–output relations in monosynaptic and poly-synaptic reflexes, to the extent that the latter are known, are illustrated in Fig. 76. Given a linear input (76A) which is essentially the case, the relation for monosynaptic reflexes (76B) is exactly that to be expected if there is a great need for summation in this pathway before discharge is realized (237). That for polysynaptic, specifically flexor, reflexes suggests that there is not the same need (76C). In these differences there lies the implication that the distribution of synaptic knobs upon motoneurones from primary afferent fibres and from interneurones may be very different. From this emerges the suggestions that monosynaptic reflex endings are scattered, possibly on various dendrites, and that internuncial endings are more clustered. Acceptance or rejection of such a notion would depend upon one's conception derived from a variety of sources as to where and how the motoneuronal discharge originates.

Note 13 (p. 17, footnote)

No one should ever lose sight of the imprecation contained in this footnote. When, for instance, one stimulates the sural nerve one stimulates the sural nerve, not merely or necessarily only the flexor reflex afferent fibres (frequently designated F.R.A.) despite the fact that the end result may be apparent only as a flexor reflex (cf. Chap. 7, p. 105).

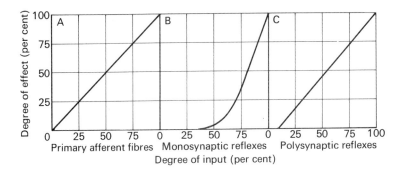

FIG. 76. A composite diagram derived from several sources to illustrate the essential difference in input-output relations of monosynaptic reflexes and polysynaptic reflexes. Fig. 76A represents the manner of recruitment of afferent fibres with increase in electrical stimulus strength. For a given group of afferent fibres the relation between stimulus strength and input is essentially linear. Fig. 76B represents the input–output curve of motoneurones to linearly incrementing monosynaptic reflex afferent impulse volleys. Fig. 76C is essentially a reitteration of the information contained in Fig. 75A. Although this last plot holds for some internuncially relayed systems that have been studied it need not necessarily hold for all.

Note 14 (p. 18, line 1)

Importance of, and indeed physiological normality of the negative afterpotential was neither realized nor recognized at the time of publication of this book. Negative afterpotential of ventral root fibres is enormous: it can cause repetitive impulses without the implication that motoneurones have discharged repetitively in response to central action. Interneurones *per contra* frequently, one might almost say usually, discharge repetitively to a single action (255).

Note 15 (p. 18, line 32 et seq.)

It is difficult to compare stimulus strengths from stimulators of one era to those of another. Who today knows what a Kronecker unit is? But from that which is now known it would certainly seem that this passage implies, by reason of increase in stimulus strength, the addition of a Group III flexor reflex to an already existing Group II flexor reflex; in other words, that the stimulus had reached delta strength. Brooks and Fuortes (213) have emphasized the change in character of the flexor reflex on increase in stimulus strength.

Note 16 (p. 21, line 11)

At the time the general concept of the reflex centre resembled that expressed diagrammatically in Fig. 77M by Lorente de Nó, which likewise resembles the 1925 diagram of Sir Charles Sherrington (188), as a multiple pathway, although the concept of circular delay paths (Forbes) or reverberating circuits (Fig. 77C) was incorporated in

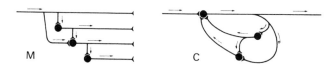

FIG. 77. Diagrams (after Lorente de Nó) of the two fundamental patterns of internuncial connexions. M, the multiple chain. C, the closed chain or reverberating circuit. Evidence of these two mechanisms at work is seen in the recordings of Fig. 78.

thinking. These concepts still hold true with respect to the flexor reflex, as can be seen in Fig. 78, which on the left shows a flexor reflex discharge with a *d'emblée* opening with 'afterdischarge' and on the right shows another flexor reflex discharge with two peaks growing the one with the other, which would not happen if the second peak were to be the consequence of recruitment of higher threshold afferent fibres into the executant afferent volley. These considerations, important as they are, have no significance with respect to mono-synaptic reflexes.

Note 17 (p. 24, line 11)

A factor not mentioned as causing increase in response during an experiment is cooling, which until recently was with time virtually inevitable. An early example of the influence of a fall in body temperature led to the discovery of the 'dorsal root reflex' (265). An example of the change in action wrought by temperature change is to be seen in Fig. 79. It concerns the response of plantar motoneurone dendrites. Two important principles are illustrated: first, some if not all neural tissue does not yield its maximal response at normal body temperature, and secondly that conduction in some neural structures is indeed decremental in character (233, 245, 260). Furthermore, inasmuch as it is coming to be generally accepted, with more evidence yet in store, that monosynaptic reflex afferent fibres terminate on dendrites, one can see that the magnitude of reflex response would be profoundly affected by the ability of dendrites to carry impulses. Monosynaptic reflexes increase with a fall in body temperature (229) and so presumably would the stretch reflex—to say nothing of other reflexes.

Note 18 (p. 37, line 12 et seq.)

Bearing in mind the nature of the flexor reflex and its anatomical substrate, together with the *c.e.s.* concept, it may be useful to emphasize the term 'nuclear delay' (232), for this rather than synaptic delay is in essence what is involved in the production of that which was called *c.e.s.* From the time when impulses begin to impinge in a given circumstance upon a nucleus until the time that impulses begin to emerge from that nucleus is the essential definition of nuclear delay. These events are directly measurable. Recognizing the concepts of Eccles and Sherrington (79, p. 579) and the nature of the flexor reflex, nuclear delay is equivalent to the time required for *c.e.s.* to reach

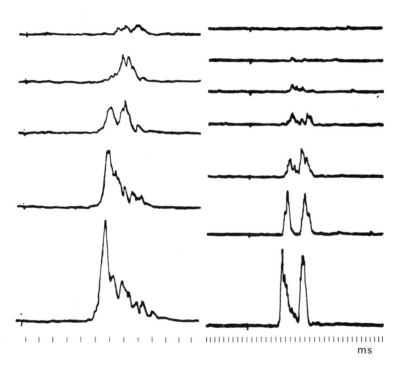

ms

FIG. 78. Flexor reflex discharges in the nerve to semitendinosus resulting (from above downwards in sequence) from incrementing single shocks to the sural nerve. On the left are typical discharges with a *d'emblée* opening and a measure of 'afterdischarge'. At the right is an example of a flexor reflex discharge similarly engendered by incrementing stimuli but with two peaks of response that grow *pari passu* with increase in stimulation strength. Because of this fact the second peak cannot be due merely to recruitment of afferent fibres but must rather represent response to a reverberating circuit.

threshold. The terms *c.e.s.* (and incidentally *c.i.s.*—the central inhibitory state—cf. Chapter VI), useful as they were, have been superseded in the course of time.

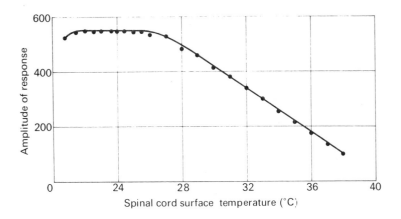

FIG. 79. Response of motoneuronal dendrites as a function of temperature. Normal temperature for the cat is approximately 38·5° C. Responses were recorded from the dorsolateral angle of the ventral horn, first sacral segment, in response to antidromic volleys to the plantar motoneurones. Temperature was measured by means of a thermocouple adjacent to the recording electrode. Dendrites of motoneurones subject to decremental conduction do not act to their full capacity at normal body temperature. Such may well be true of numerous other neural elements.

Note 19 (p. 38, line 4)

Temporal dispersion of reflex discharge no longer is considered a result of differences in 'synaptic' delays at different motoneurones. The logical concept including the notion of delays amounting to 6 or 8 ms derives from the *c.e.s.* hypothesis. This critical comment should not be construed as denying that such delays may occur at certain loci. At the present time they are not known to exist. Such difficulty as there may be derives from the changed concept of synaptic delay (with respect to fixity and brevity) consequent upon direct electrical recording of neuronal activity. Hence lies, in part, utility of the term 'nuclear delay' in relation to growth of *c.e.s.* to threshold value.

Note 20 (p. 38, line 28 – p. 42, line 7)

The entire subject of effects of antidromic volleys into motoneurones has become so complex that it cannot be dealt with in a reasonable space (cf. 214, 233, 238, 245, 252, 259, 260). But it can be noted that an antidromic volley to the motoneurones reveals that the absolutely refractory period of the soma is 1·5 ms, approximately 1 ms longer than that of the axones; that the relative refractory period is in duration from 7 to 10 ms in agreement with earlier measurements presented in this chapter, and that it is followed by a subnormal period some 120 ms in duration, which presumably accounts for the observation that an 'antidromic volley . . . must inactivate some of the *c.e.s.*' (p. 41, line 14).

Note 21 (p. 42, line 9)

After-discharge presents a difficult problem if for no other reason than that today no one knows how it should be defined. Much of the motor discharge seen in Fig. 74B or Fig. 78 could be called after-discharge. But the strict definition would regard after-discharge as a discharge of nerve impulses by nerve cells as the result of the arrival of presynaptic nerve impulses but not dependent upon the continued arrival of such impulses. In this strict sense the continued discharge of the flexor reflex could not be called after-discharge. True after-discharge would call, as stated on p. 42, line 11 'for a prolonged excitatory condition at some part of the central reflex pathway'. Some interneurones unquestionably respond repetitively at frequencies initially as high at 1000 Hz to a single afferent action (255). At the motoneurone there is beyond 15 ms no such prolonged condition known, and this condition has not been seen to give rise to and apparently is incapable of giving rise to repetitive response (214). The prolonged response in Fig. 78 is relatable to continued activity by interneurones. Adopting a loose definition of after-discharge it is in the flexor reflex related largely to increase in strength of stimulation that brings impingement upon the motoneurones the consequences of stimulation of Group III (delta) afferent fibres (213, 234, 239, 244) although there is asynchronous response to Group II volleys. Block of 'after-discharge' by an antidromic volley is due to interposition of a subnormal period in the motoneurone somata by that volley.

Note 22 (p. 46, line 2)

At this juncture it is appropriate to make a summary of the 'excitatory state' as it appears at the present time from the study of monosynaptic reflex systems. By the use of a weak conditioning shock, encompassing but a fraction of the Group IA afferent fibres of one head of a muscle, and a test stimulus which can be maximal to the afferent fibres of the other head (as in gastrocnemius medialis and lateralis), and recording from the appropriate ventral root, it is found that the response of the tested motoneurones is maximally facilitated when the conditioning and test volleys are synchronous. As the two volleys are separated in time, response to the test volley declines exponentially to $1/e$ in

about 4 ms and reaches its control value in approximately 15 ms. Fig.
80 illustrates the course of monosynaptic reflex facilitation (*c.e.s.*) in
an extensor and in a flexor nucleus respectively. These are the changes
in excitability that occur without intervention of internuncial activity
and are identical in flexor and extensor motor nuclei. These excitability changes can be correlated with an excitatory postsynaptic
potential (214) usually abbreviated as e.p.s.p.

At this point opinions differ strongly. Some would hold that the
monosynaptic e.p.s.p. gives rise to the monosynaptic reflex (cf. 214).

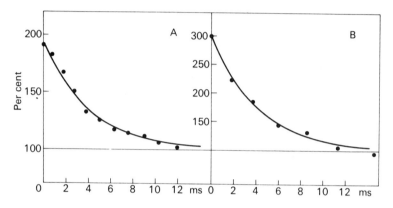

FIG. 80. Monosynaptic reflex facilitation of monosynaptic reflexes.
A, conditioning of motoneurones to one head of triceps surae by weak
Group I afferent volleys from the other head (extensor). B, conditioning
of motoneurones to biceps femoris posterior by weak Group I afferent
volleys from its synergist semitendinosus (flexor).

Others, mindful of the dual nature of the membrane potential of nerve
tissue, feel that the e.p.s.p. has the quality of an afterpotential and
that it can be responsible for facilitation both spatial and temporal but
not for monosynaptic reflex discharge (239, 246, 247). To the latter
it is the Q-fraction of Lorente de Nó (251) that is related to monosynaptic reflex discharge and, except at virtual simultaneity, it is the
L-fraction change that serves for the longer course of facilitation in
this simplest reflex arc.

Temporal facilitation follows the same time course as does spatial
facilitation (cf. Fig. 80) in the monosynaptic pathway, which is to say
that it can be described by an exponential curve decaying to $1/e$ in
4 ms (241).

Importance attaches to the questions of fixity and brevity of synaptic
delay. Fixity is now generally accepted although the value given varies
according to conceptual approaches and the measurements of collateral

conduction time one accepts (cf. 247). The *c.e.s.* hypothesis would permit of very long 'synaptic delays', but Sherrington specifically stated that each increment of *c.e.s.* would be caused by the arrival at the motoneurone of additional impulses. Hence the reason for introduction of the term 'nuclear delay' to distinguish between synaptic delay as now understood and the time taken as in a flexor reflex for an input to secure an output; otherwise, to bring *c.e.s.* to threshold. At the heart of the overall question is the duration of the presynaptic event that causes postsynaptic response. This is best shown in an experiment by Hunt (229). Fig. 81 exemplifies the result.

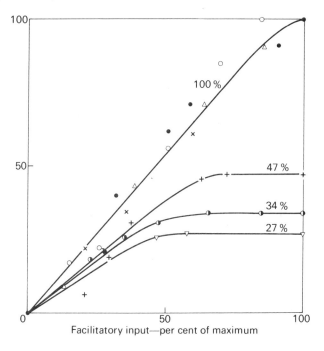

FIG. 81. Relation between the degree of monosynaptic reflex facilitation of afferent volleys from one head of triceps surae varied in strength from zero to maximum and the size of text volleys in the other head fixed at various sizes as indicated. Ordinates—growth of facilitation. Abscissae—measured conditioning input.

The term 'synchronous volley' is useful, but except at the cathode of a pair of stimulating electrodes it is an euphemism. It usually loosely implies a single volley of impulses that has not suffered much dispersion. The band of fibres afferent for the monosynaptic reflexes extends in diameter from approximately 14 to 21 μm (258). Given in approximation a relation between velocity and diameter, a volley engendered by a single shock must suffer a degree of dispersion. Given a relation between threshold and diameter it follows that a lesser stimulus will stimulate a fraction of the fibres that would be included in response to a greater stimulus and that *ceteris paribus* this fraction will consist of largest diameter and highest velocity members of the group. Thus dispersion of the consequent volley in them must be less than dispersion of that pertaining to the group as a whole.

If a conditioning volley in the afferent fibres from one head of gastrocnemius is caused to converge synchronously with another but maximal Group I afferent volley from the other head of gastrocnemius then it is found that the motoneurone response to the latter (testing) volley increments in virtually linear relation to magnitude of the varying conditioning volley (Fig. 81, curve 100 per cent).

When the test volley is reduced to 47 per cent of maximum, the conditioning volley varying as before, it is found that response to the test volley fails to increment once the conditioning volley reaches approximately 65 per cent of its maximum. As the test volley is further reduced, failure of the conditioning volley to cause increment in response to the test volley occurs at progressively lower fractions of the total test volley input. This can only mean that even with the use of quite reasonably synchronized impulses the earlier cannot sum with the later to secure discharge by the motoneurones and hence that the transmitting ability of presynaptic impulses at the motoneurone is extremely brief. According to Hunt (229) it has decayed significantly within 0·2–0·3 ms. It is probably confined to the alteration phase of the impinging presynaptic impulses (251). This phase is extremely brief but the fact itself does not preclude adoption of either an electrical or of a chemical hypothesis of transmission according to predilection.

Note 23 (p. 46, line 7)

The mechanism of summation from different synapses is still not clear. However it is known that the space constant of the transmitting effect (229, 237, 252), as differentiated from the facilitating agent, is so short in the somata of motoneurones that the action of some synaptic knobs (*boutons*) need not, indeed do not, sum with the action of some others impinging upon the same motoneurone. This observation, of course, is another stumbling-block in the way of considering the e.p.s.p. as the cause of motoneurone discharge, for the e.p.s.p. is generally considered to encompass the entire motoneuronal soma (cell body and dendrites).

It is germane to add that the wavelength of an action potential in the soma is extremely short by comparison with that in nerve fibres (252). For a given value of membrane potential change during an impulse, for example, current flow about somata is much more intense

than that about nerve-fibres, all lying within the volume conductor
which is the spinal cord. This in turn accounts for the much larger
responses recorded by an extracellular microelectrode placed in the
region of a nucleus than those recorded by similar means from fibre
tracts (247).

IV. THE STRETCH REFLEX

Note 24 (p. 50, line 16)

The history of study of the tendon-jerk is a fascinating subject.
Reference here is made initially to the shortest possible phasic reaction
which has very nearly the time dimensions of an unitary spike potential

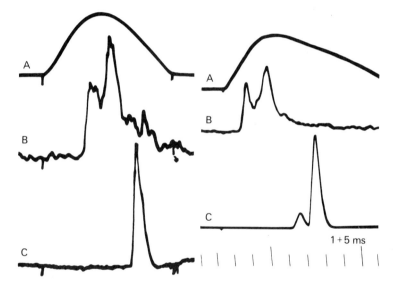

FIG. 82. Stretch reflexes. Recordings on the left and on the right are in
general similar. In each instance record A represents the course of pull,
photoelectrically recorded, upon the tendon of triceps surae. Record B in
each case records from the first sacral dorsal root the afferent response to the
respective pulls. Record C in each case illustrates the reflex response to the
respective afferent activity documented in the records B.

in nerve. On the left side of Fig. 82 record A plots the time course of
pull on the tendon of triceps surae. Record B shows the afferent fibre
response to an identical pull. There are two main afferent volleys
followed by some more asynchronous activity. The first of these
afferent volleys proved to be subliminal at the motoneurones. The

second, facilitated by the first, gave rise to the reflex response seen recorded from a ventral root in record C. This response secured by natural stimulation has the time dimensions of a monosynaptic reflex elicited by electrical stimulation of the afferent nerve. Frequently the first afferent volley evoked by stretch is successful in securing a reflex discharge, as seen on the right of Fig. 82. When this happens the motor discharge resulting from brief stretch consists typically of two synchronized motor volleys as in the lowermost record to the right of Fig. 82. The second motor volley undoubtedly was facilitated by the subliminal fringe of the first (235). The later afferent activity seen in record B on both the left and right halves of Fig. 82 apparently in terms of motor expression suffers the consequence of subnormality induced in the motoneurones by its predecessors.

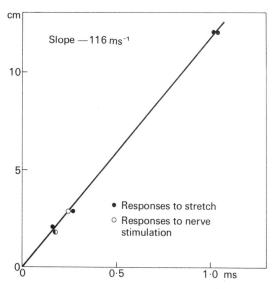

FIG. 83. Comparison of the conduction velocity of afferent impulses in response to stretch of triceps surae with that of afferent impulses engendered by electrical stimulation of the nerve. Responses were recorded from two points on the afferent pathway and the latency of the two sorts of response plotted against conduction distance.

Note 25 (p. 51, line 12)

Conduction velocity of stretch reflex afferent fibres is now known to approximate 120 m/s, and is at that value equal to the velocity of the most rapidly conducting afferent fibres in the muscle nerve (Fig. 83).

Although this is a higher figure than that given, nevertheless the calculations all fit and there is no doubt, for this reason *inter alia*, that the monosynaptic reflex is in effect the electrically stimulated equivalent of the tendon-jerk. Whether the sustained or 'static reaction' reflex depends only on this monosynaptic reflex structure is open to question. It might be imprudent to suppose that it is.

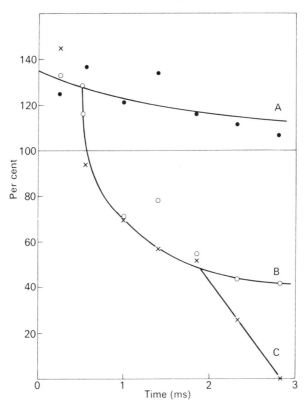

FIG. 84. Conditioning action upon test monosynaptic reflexes of plantaris (extensor) of graded afferent volleys in the nerve of its flexor antagonist flexor digitorum longus. A, weak (IA) afferent volleys. B, stronger (IA + IB) afferent volleys. C, still stronger (Group I + Group II) volleys in the conditioning nerve.

Note 26 (p. 54, line 36)

Weak stimulation of Group I afferent fibres yields a facilitation curve of response in a synergist as shown in Fig. 80 and in curve A of Fig. 84 (230). A slight increase in conditioning stimulus strength will result in the change indicated by Fig. 84, curve B. The divergence from pure facilitation occurs abruptly at a stimulus interval of 0·5 ms. As the conditioning stimulus strength is in the Group I range this can only mean that Group IB fibres had been recruited into the afferent volleys confined by the weaker stimulus to Group IA fibres. It is generally conceded that Group IA fibres arise in the muscle-spindles and serve for the stretch reflex. Likewise it is generally conceded that Group IB fibres arise in tendon organs. Thus on the basis of physiological evidence the latter mediate the 'lengthening reaction', which is the counter to the stretch reflex. Further increase in strength of stimulus produced the curve of Fig. 84C. At this strength Group II fibres were stimulated and the abrupt change at 2 ms separation of stimuli, the nucleus under study being an extensor nucleus, represents the inhibitory component of the flexor reflex.

Thus the myotatic reflex and the lengthening reaction are mediated by the same band with lesser or greater but always small difference in threshold to electrical stimulation (Fig. 84). When seeking the differences between monosynaptic and disynaptic reflexes on the one hand and between stretch reflexes and the lengthening reaction on the other, we must take account of the fact that in one instance we are dealing with electrical stimulation of bared nerves and in the other with natural stimulation affected by the action of afferent end organs. In part at least, the results of Laporte and Lloyd (230) can be accounted for by the elegant experiment of Sumner (Fig. 85) (cf. 254, Fig. 1). Sumner isolated single afferent fibres in the nerve to triceps surae, measuring nerve threshold for each fibre, determining its conduction velocity, and defining its receptor of origin. By relating the threshold of each unit to the threshold and Group I maximal stimulation of the entire nerve in each instance he was able to plot the pooled results from the individual fibres. Thus the unit thresholds could be related to the overall growth of the Group I volley with respect to stimulus strength. If Group IA and Group IB thresholds were evenly distributed the points for both sorts would lie on the broken line in Fig. 85. But the points for Group IA fibres lie well above and those for Group IB well below the broken line. This difference then is one reason why the reflex result illustrated in Fig. 84 could have been obtained. It is of interest to compare these findings with those contained in Fig. 73.

An additional difference is that afferent impulses of the myotatic reflex are delivered directly to the motoneurones, whereas those mediating the lengthening reaction (autogenetic inhibition or inverse myotatic reflex) have an interneurone interposed in their pathway to the motoneurone.

There may not be enough difference in the two sorts of afferent fibres to account for the physiological differences between the two reflexes in the decerebrate preparation. Inhibition of the lengthening reaction, rather than excitation of the stretch reflex, predominates in the spinal preparation, unless one is dealing with highly synchronized

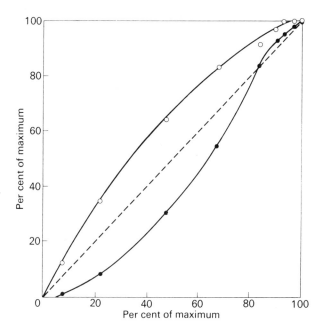

FIG. 85. Group I volleys are very nearly linearly related to strength of stimulation. However Group IA fibres are biased slightly to the greater diameter (and hence lower threshold) members of the group, whereas Group IB fibres are slightly biased toward the lower diametre members (cf. Fig. 73). This figure shows how in terms of threshold the two subgroups vary as a Group I volley progresses from zero to maximum.

brief stretch in which case the excitatory impulses arrive first in time and so gain temporary ascendency.

That stretch excitation of autochthonous motoneurones is present at all degrees of stretch follows from the fact that monosynapticity of action implies inevitability of action. This is true to the extent that action is not after a while modified by so-called presynaptic inhibition caused by some neurones depressing the action of some presynaptic fibres by virtue of synapsis with them (218, 219). That inhibition may dominate in the spinal state and yet be held in check (up to a certain level of stretch) undoubtedly means that the internuncial link in the disynaptic or lengthening reflex path is open in the spinal preparation and up to a crucial level of stretch closed in the decerebrate. This is the action of a valve (242).[1] There may well be collateral to the stretch reflex afferent fibres (Group IA) a connexion, inhibitory in character, to the interneurones of the lengthening reflex pathway which holds the latter in obeyance until such time as the input from tendon organs becomes overwhelming. For these two responses to stretch to be co-ordinated appropriately it would seem essential that interneurones known to exist should act as a 'shut-off' valve in the pathway for the lengthening reaction.

The foregoing also raises the question of higher centres controlling afferent input, a question put in 1944 and much enlarged upon in recent years (but cf. 262).

Note 27 (p. 56, line 5)

The silent period is a little more complicated in its mechanism than had been supposed. There is, of course, the slackening of strain on the muscle-spindles here referred to. There is also the inhibitory component demonstrated by Denny-Brown (62), which corresponds to the inverse myotatic reflex illustrated in Fig. 84. But there is, in addition, the subnormal period of the motoneurones (238) that had not yet been discovered, following upon their discharge. It lasts for some 120 ms. Furthermore, this cause for silence would not necessarily be limited to the discharged motoneurones, for motoneurone discharge can depress the excitability of neighbouring motoneurones either by current flows or through the action of recurrent collaterals depending upon one's point of view. Thus this action may be added to the inhibition shown by Denny-Brown (62) to be present to account for a silent period occurring in motor units other than those discharged in the tendon-jerk.

Group IA and Group IB endings, as is now obvious, behave in opposite senses. A particularly clear demonstration of this is contained in experiments by Hunt (239 — after Hunt) illustrated in Fig. 86. At the top left is the resting discharge of a Group IA (spindle) single afferent fibre under slight stretch and just below it is the essentially quiet myogram. At the lower left is seen in the myographic record the course of tension change in a single twitch and in the electrogram cessation of spindle afferent fibre discharge during contraction and the slight increase in frequency of discharge during relaxation. This part of Fig. 86 should be compared with Fig. 23 in the original text.

[1] With respect to reflex transmission Sherrington employed the word 'valve' to imply something that permits passage in one direction but not in its reverse (the doctrine of forward direction). As used here the word implies something (such as a cut-off valve) that either allows or prevents some result depending upon whether or not it is open.

At the right of Fig. 86 at the top, recorded in similar circumstances but with a single Group IB fibre on the recording electrodes, is seen the quiescent myogram and electrogram. At the right below is recorded an identical muscle twitch accompanied by a burst of activity in the Group IB (tendon organ) fibre.

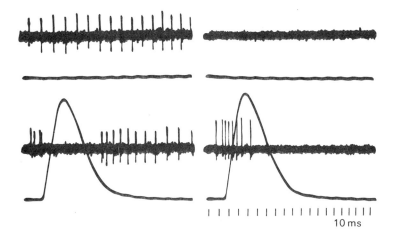

10 ms

FIG. 86. Response of A (spindle) and B (tendon organ) type afferent endings in muscle. Afferent response and muscle tension are recorded simultaneously and appear as the wider and finer lines respectively in each record pair. Top left, steadily maintained A-type discharge, the result of weak stretch. Bottom left, cessation of A-type discharge during twitch contraction and slight discharge rebound. Compare with Fig. 23. Top right, there is no sustained discharge of B-type ending at the degree of stretch imposed. Bottom right, discharge of B-type ending during active twitch contraction. Original experiment by C. C. Hunt.

V. REFLEXES IN EXTENSOR MUSCLES OTHER THAN POSTURAL REFLEXES

Relatively little has been done with which to supplement this chapter. The outstanding exception has been the work of Perl on crossed reflex action (256–8). A brief description of it follows. In these papers Perl studied crossed effects caused by stimulation of cutaneous nerves, of muscle nerves, and by muscle stretch. Many of his observations might well be described in relation to the content of p. 73, line 7 *et seq.* He has made use of the distinctions between the fibre constitution of cutaneous and muscular afferent fibres (Fig. 72) and of those between Group IA (spindle) and Group IB (Golgi tendon organs) fibres (Figs. 73 and 85) in the course of his analyses.

A volley in cutaneous Group II afferent fibres facilitates the action of crossed knee and ankle flexors with a short latency (c. 3 ms). Sometimes extensors were inhibited. On increasing stimulus strength to include Group III afferent fibres in the volley a prolonged inhibition of crossed flexors followed the initial facilitation. This was coupled with facilitation of the crossed extensors (256). Here is evidence that Group III afferent fibres are concerned with the crossed extensor reflex.

On stimulating muscle afferent fibres Perl found that the Group I afferent fibres of a given muscle inhibited and then facilitated action of the corresponding muscle on the contralateral side. Inhibition appeared to be related to action of the IA spindle afferent fibres and so would be reciprocal with respect to the stretch reflex whereas excitation appeared to be related to action of IB tendon afferent fibres and so related reciprocally to the lengthening reaction. Group II afferent fibres of muscle were inhibitory to crossed flexor muscles. Recruitment of Group III muscle afferent fibres produced facilitation in knee flexors of the opposite side. But within 20 to 30 ms such a volley, whether arising from flexor or extensor muscles, caused facilitation of both knee and ankle extensor motoneurones lasting for some 100 ms (257).

A small stretch applied to either a flexor or extensor (258) caused inhibition of the motoneurones of the homonymous crossed muscle. Stronger pull caused inhibition to give way to facilitation. Again the presumption is that IA fibres yield crossed inhibition as a circumscribed concomitant of the stretch reflex and that IB fibres yield a crossed concomitant of the lengthening reaction.

Obviously there is an admixture of crossed reflex effect (cf. Chap. VII, p. 107), but it is equally clear that the crossed extensor reflex must arise in the tendon organs and from other receptors that play upon the smaller afferent fibres, notably Group III. Therefore the crossed extensor reflex is, in terms of reciprocal innervation, undoubtedly a complex affair, in part a concomitant of the inverse myotatic reflex (the lengthening reaction) and also of certain (notably Group III) ipsilateral flexor reflexes.

Altogether there would appear to be at least three reflex entities when the full range of contralateral afferent fibres is stimulated.

VI. CENTRAL INHIBITION

With the advent of direct electronic recording from roots, nerves, and central neurones, and the unequivocal demonstration of monosynaptic reflexes, the possibility of examining inhibition in the same manner as facilitation (Fig. 80) at the motoneurone arose once an example of direct inhibition had been found (231, 235). It was found initially in dorsal to ventral root preparations (231) and its functional significance was not immediately appreciated. Soon it was noted that the afferent fibres responsible for this simple form of inhibition were indistinguishable from those executant for monosynaptic reflexes (Fig. 87). Later direct inhibition was found to be confined to the

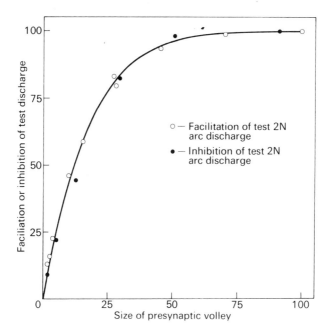

FIG. 87. A comparison between the development of monosynaptic reflex excitation and monosynaptic reflex inhibition in intensity with respect to increase in size of conditioning afferent volleys engendered in appropriate dorsal roots. The shape of the curve is determined in part by the fact that the higher threshold fibres in a dorsal root do not contribute to monosynaptic reflex action. Nevertheless it is obvious that the excitatory and inhibitory monosynaptic reflex fibres are indistinguishable.

antagonists of any given muscle to which the monosynaptic myotatic reflex discharge was directed. It is, in fact, the reciprocally related inhibitory component of the tendon jerk (or pluck reflex), whether instigated from flexor or extensor muscle Group I afferent fibres.

Fig. 88 illustrates the time course of inhibition caused by small

(i.e. Group IA) afferent volleys: in 88A of tibialis anterior motoneurones (flexor) by volleys from triceps surae (extensor) and in
88B of triceps surae motoneurones by volleys in the deep peroneal
nerve. The course of direct inhibition is identical in flexor and

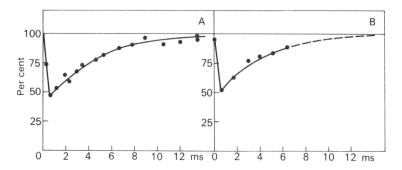

FIG. 88. A, monosynaptic reflex inhibition of tibialis anterior (flexor)
monosynaptic reflexes by Group IA afferent volleys from the nerve to triceps surae (the extensor antagonist). B, Monosynaptic reflex inhibition by
Group IA volleys in the nerve of triceps surae (extensor) upon the monosynaptic reflex to the deep pereoneal nerve (representing ankle flexors and
digital dorsiflexors). The course of monosynaptic reflex inhibition is
identical in flexor and extensor nuclei.

extensor motoneurone pools and in its decay is identical with that of
monosynaptic reflex facilitation (Fig. 80).

An inhibitory postsynaptic potential roughly paralleling that of
monosynaptic reflex inhibition has been described (214). It is cus-
tomarily displayed by the use of an intracellular microelectrode
placed within a motoneurone. Its mechanism, normality, and latency
are controversial (247, 250), but the fact that it occurs suggests
a revision of the thought expressed on p. 103, line 1 that *c.i.s.* has no
direct effect upon the motoneurone.

Some would maintain that the i.p.s.p., as the inhibitory potential
is abbreviated, is the agent for inhibition—others demur. Sufficient to
say at the present time that reliance upon its manifestations for critical
measurements such as latency may be frought with danger (247).

Great emphasis has been placed upon 'Dale's principle', to the
effect that if a neurone liberates a given transmitter substance at some
of its terminals it is likely to liberate the same transmitter at all of its
terminals. If it is considered that separate transmitters are requisite
for excitation and inhibition then some transferral mechanism must
be postulated to produce in the Group IA pathway an inhibitory
substance to act upon antagonist motoneurones. From one point of
view an interneurone is considered to be intercallated in the Group

IA inhibitory pathway to achieve this end. This postulated inter-neurone when excited would produce a different (inhibitory) trans-mitter at the motoneurones (214).

There are two major objections to the foregoing concept. The first is that in some instances one and the same transmitter has been found to have opposite effects, excitatory and inhibitory, upon a single neurone, depending presumably upon differences in the postsynaptic membrane at different loci, thus obviating the necessity for invoking an interneurone to satisfy Dale's principle.

The experimental finding related above does not violate Dale's principle but it prompts a quotation from Sir Charles Sherrington written in 1925 (188): 'Cytological evidence as well as physiological consideration teaches that the perikaryon substance presents differences (of staining, etc.), from point to point. For the terminal *boutons* themselves evidence of such differentiation one from another is strikingly lacking. These data suggest that two terminals, though themselves essentially similar, may yet act in the perikaryon on subsurface material of different kinds, so that one may cause there an excitatory, the other an inhibitory response. Separate intracentral terminals of one and the same (e.g. afferent) nerve-fibre may thus produce in some of them excitation response in perikarya they reach, while others in other perikarya produce inhibitional response.' If he had not established so many other principles the foregoing might well be called 'Sherrington's principle'. There exists abundant evidence that this principle harmonizes with the experimental facts subsequently disclosed both histological and physiological (231, 236, 247, 250, 263). Furthermore, it neither conflicts with nor nullifies Dale's principle.

The second objection to the concept of an intercalated inter-neurone in the Group IA inhibitory pathway to motoneurones is that time relations as now understood would not allow of its presence (216, 247, 250). Clearly such a controversial subject, despite convictions, requires time and experimental effort for its resolution.

Much attention recently has been accorded to recurrent inhibition (lateral inhibition). In one form or another it has been encountered in many places within the nervous system. In specific reference to the spinal cord, it was first noted by Renshaw (259). Interestingly, it accounts for the inhibition that Sherrington found in one head of a muscle upon stimulation of the nerve to another head (169, 170). In this case, as in that later observed by Renshaw, the inhibition proves to have been an antidromic phenomenon. Full details concerning this action are to be found in Eccles' monograph (214), but it is worth-while reiterating that an antidromic volley imposes a subnormal period upon those motoneurones it penetrates and cannot do other-wise than influence their responsivity. Thus if *c.e.s.* were to be in a motoneurone it would be affected by an antidromic volley. But if *c.i.s.* inactivates *c.e.s.*, the latter being in the motoneurone, then it must have an effect upon or be in the motoneurone (p. 103, line 1).

Antidromic volleys induce facilitation in some motoneurones as first observed by Renshaw (259). This facilitation is now considered to be an inhibition of tonic inhibitory activity (226, 266)—in effect a 'disinhibition'.

Another phenomenon that has attracted much attention recently is that called 'presynaptic inhibition' (214, 218, 219), or 'remote inhibition'. It is said to result from the action of axo-axonic synapses whereby the action of the receiving afferent fibres is reduced. The fundamental observation underlying this concept is the occurrence of depression in a motoneurone without concomitant recordable production of an inhibitory postsynaptic potential (218). Presynaptic inhibition is temporally similar, but not necessarily causally related, to the dorsal root potential of Barron and Matthews (210) and thus in a way to the positive cord potential of Gasser and Graham (224) and of Hughes and Gasser (227, 228). The entire subject of presynaptic inhibition is in a state of flux. One needs to know if the i.p.s.p. is a significant reality or an artefact consequent upon experimental procedures. Then, if it is a physiological reality, is it produced, as considered by Frank (218), so far out on the dendrites in the instance of presynaptic inhibition that it might not be seen by an intracellular microelectrode? Hence the use by Frank of the term 'remote inhibition'. All one can say at the present time is that opinions differ.

Note 28 (p. 93, Fig. 49)

This intriguing effect illustrated remains to the present time not fully explained. Considering the duration of antagonist inhibition within a myotatic unit (Fig. 88) one can only suppose that the conditioning single shock involved Group III and possibly C fibres for there to have been such enduring inhibition of knee jerks by a single shock to the nerve of the antagonist.

Note 29 (p. 102, line 25)

Experimental evidence has now documented amply the occurrence of inhibition at neurones other than motoneurones (214).

Note 30 (p. 103, line 1 et seq.)

Except for the examples of 'presynaptic inhibition' and for the inhibition of interneurones it is no longer held that inhibitory action has no direct effect upon the motoneurone.

VII. LOWER REFLEX CO-ORDINATION

On study of this chapter one comes to realize to what great extent advances made since its inception concern mechanism and that the overall picture of reflex taxis remains virtually as Sir Charles Sherrington and his colleagues left it. In other words, the spinal machinery is somewhat different from that which had been envisaged but the end result of its action is the same.

REFERENCES

1. ADLER, F. H. (1930). 'Reciprocal innervation of the extraocular muscles.' *Arch. Ophthal.* **3**, 318.
2. ADRIAN, E. D. (1926). 'The impulses produced by sensory nerve endings.' *J. Physiol.* **61**, 49.
3. —— (1926). 'The impulses produced by sensory nerve endings. Part 4. Impulses from pain receptors.' *J. Physiol.* **62**, 33.
4. —— (1928). *The Basis of Sensation.* London.
5. —— (1930). 'The mechanism of the sense organs.' *Physiol. Rev.* **10**, 336.
6. —— (1930). 'The effects of injury on mammalian nerve-fibres.' *Proc. Roy. Soc.* **106** B, 596.
7. ADRIAN, E. D., McK. CATTELL, and H. HOAGLAND (1931). 'Response of tactile receptors to intermittent stimulation.' *J. Physiol.* **72**, 392.
8. ADRIAN, E. D., and A. FORBES (1922). 'The all-or-nothing response of sensory nerve-fibres.' *J. Physiol.* **56**, 301.
9. ADRIAN, E. D., and Y. ZOTTERMAN (1926). 'The impulses produced by sensory nerve endings.' *J. Physiol.* **61**, 151.
10. ADRIAN, E. D., and D. W. BRONK (1928, 1929). 'The discharge of impulses in motor-nerve-fibres. I. Impulses in single fibres of the phrenic nerve.' *J. Physiol.* **66**, 81. 'II. Frequency of discharge in reflex and voluntary contractions.' *J. Physiol.* **67**, 119.
11. ADRIAN, E. D., and H. UMRATH (1929). 'The impulse discharge from the Pacinian corpuscle.' *J. Physiol.* **68**, 139.
12. ADRIAN, E. D., and F. J. J. BUYTENDIJK (1931). 'Potential changes in the isolated brain-stem of the goldfish.' *J. Physiol.* **71**, 121.
13. ASAYAMA, C. (1915). 'The proprioceptive reflex of a flexor muscle.' *Quart. J. Exp. Physiol.* **9**, 265.

14. BALLIF, L., J. F. FULTON, and E. G. T. LIDDELL (1925). 'Observations on spinal and decerebrate knee-jerks with special reference to their inhibition by single break-shocks.' *Proc. Roy. Soc.* **98** B, 589.
15. BAYLISS, W. M. (1924). *Principles of General Physiology.* London
16. BAZETT, H. C., and W. G. PENFIELD (1922). 'A study of the Sherrington decerebrate animal in the chronic as well as the acute condition.' *Brain*, **45**, 185.
17. BERITOFF, J. S. (1915). 'On the mode of origination of labyrinthine and cervical tonic reflexes and their part in the reflex reactions of the decerebrate preparation.' *Quart. J. Exp. Physiol.* **9**, 199.
18. —— (1924). 'Über den Rhythmus der reziproken Innervation

198   REFERENCES

der antagonistischen Muskeln bei Warmblütern.' *Z. Biol.* **80** 171.

19. BERNSTEIN, J. (1912). 'Electrobiologie.' Braunschweig.

20. BISHOP, G. H., and P. HEINBECKER (1930). 'Differentiation of axon types in visceral nerves by means of the potential record.' *Amer. J. Physiol.* **94**, 170.

21. BOZLER, E. (1927). 'Untersuchungen über das Nervensystem der Coelenteraten.' *Z. Zellforsch. Mik. Anat.* **5**, 244.

22. BREMER, F. (1923). 'Physiologie nerveuse de la mastication chez le chat et le lapin.' *Arch. int. Physiol.* **21**, 309.

23. —— (1925). 'Recherches sur le mécanisme de l'action de la strychnine sur le système nerveux.' *Arch. int. Physiol.* **25**, 131.

24. —— (1929). 'Nouvelles recherches sur la sommation d'influx nerveux.' *C. R. Soc. Biol. Paris*, **102**, 332.

25. —— (1930). 'La sommation d'influx nerveux dans l'arc réflexe spinal.' *C. R. Soc. Biol. Paris*, **103**, 509.

26. —— (1930). 'De la période réfractaire de l'arc réflexe spinal.' *C. R. Soc. Biol. Paris*, **103**, 513.

27. —— (1930). 'Nouvelles recherches sur la sommation centrale.' *C. R. Soc. Biol. Paris*, **104**, 810.

28. —— (1931). 'Contributions à l'étude du phénomène de l'inhibition centrale.' *C. R. Soc. Biol. Paris*, **106**, 465.

29. BREMER, F., and P. RYLANT (1924). 'Action de la strychnine sur l'excitabilité des différents éléments de l'arc réflexe.' *C. R. Soc. Biol. Paris*, **91**, 110.

30. ——, —— (1925). 'Nouvelles recherches sur le mécanisme de l'action de la strychnine sur le système nerveux central.' *C. R. Soc. Biol. Paris*, **92**, 199.

31. ——, —— (1925). 'L'action locale de la strychnine sur les nerfs et les centres.' *C. R. Soc. Biol. Paris*, **92**, 1329.

32. BREMER, F., and G. HOMÈS (1931). 'Une théorie de la sommation d'influx nerveux.' *Mém. Acad. Roy. Belg.*, **11**, fasc. 7.

33. BRONK, D. W. (1930). 'The energy expended in maintaining a muscular contraction.' *J. Physiol.* **69**, 306.

34. BROWN, T. GRAHAM (1911). 'Studies in the physiology of the nervous system. IX.' *Quart. J. Exp. Physiol.* **4**, 332.

35. —— (1911). 'The intrinsic factors in the act of progression in the mammal.' *Proc. Roy. Soc.* **84**, 308.

36. —— (1912). 'The factors in rhythmic activity of the nervous system.' *Proc. Roy. Soc.* **85** B, 278.

37. —— (1913). 'The phenomenon of "Narcosis Progression" in mammals.' *Proc. Roy. Soc.* **86** B, 140.

38. —— (1914). 'On the nature of the fundamental activity of the nervous centres; together with an analysis of rhythmic activity.' *J. Physiol.* **48**, 18.

39. —— (1924). 'Studies in the physiology of the nervous system. XXVIII.' *Quart. J. Exp. Physiol.* **14**, 1.

REFERENCES   199

40. BROWN, T. GRAHAM (1927). 'Upon inhibitory relaxations evoked
    by reflex stimuli of constant intensity acting against varied
    magnitudes of extensor tone.' *J. Physiol.* **63**, 197.
41. —— (1927). 'The relation of the magnitudes of remaining reflex
    shortening in two antagonistic muscles during compound
    stimulation.' *Proc. Roy. Soc.* **102**, 159.
42. BROWN, T. GRAHAM, and C. S. SHERRINGTON (1912). 'The rule
    of reflex response in the limb reflexes of the mammal and its
    exceptions.' *J. Physiol.* **44**, 125.
    BRÜCKE, E. T. *See* von Brücke, E. T.
43. BUYTENDIJK, F. J. J. (1912). 'Über die elektrischen Erscheinungen
    bei der reflektorischen Innervation der Skelettmuskulatur
    des Säugetieres.' *Z. Biol.* **59**, 35.

44. CAJAL, S. R. (1909). *Histologie du Système Nerveux*, **1**, 313.
    Paris.
45. CAMIS, M. (1909). 'On the unity of motor centres.' *J. Physiol.*
    39, 228.
46. CHARLET, H. (1930). 'Fortgesetzte Untersuchungen über den Ein-
    fluss des Sympathikus auf den Kontraptionsablauf ermüdeter
    Skelettmuskeln.' *Z. Biol.* **90**, 299 (from laboratory of Prof.
    L. Asher).
47. CHAUVEAU, A. (1891). 'On the sensori-motor nerve-circuit of
    muscle.' *Brain*, **14**, 145.
48. CLARK, D. A. (1930). 'Muscle counts of motor units.' *J. Physiol.*
    70, xviii.
    —— (1931). 'Muscle counts of motor units.—A study in
    innervation ratios.' *Amer. J. Physiol.* **96**, 296.
49. COOPER, S. (1929). 'The relation of active to inactive fibres in
    fractional contraction of muscle.' *J. Physiol.* **67**, 1.
50. COOPER, S., and E. D. ADRIAN (1924). 'The electric response in
    reflex contractions of spinal and decerebrate preparations.'
    Proc. Roy. Soc. **96** B, 243.
51. COOPER, S., D. E. DENNY BROWN, and C. S. SHERRINGTON
    (1926). 'Reflex fractionation of a muscle.' *Proc. Roy. Soc.*
    100 B, 448.
52. ——, ——, —— (1927). 'Interaction between ipselateral spinal
    reflexes acting on the flexor muscles of the hind limb.' *Proc.*
    Roy. Soc. **101** B, 262.
53. COOPER, S., and R. S. CREED (1927). 'Reflex effects of active
    muscular contraction.' *J. Physiol.* **62**, 273.
54. COOPER, S., and D. E. DENNY BROWN (1927). 'Responses to
    stimulation of the motor area of the cerebral cortex.' *Proc.*
    Roy. Soc. **102** B, 222.
55. COOPER, S., and R. S. CREED (1928). 'More reflex effects of
    active muscular contraction.' *J. Physiol.* **64**, 199.
56. COOPER, S., and D. E. DENNY BROWN (1929). 'The interaction

between two trains of impulses converging on the same motoneurone.' *Proc. Roy. Soc.* **105** B, 363.

57. COOPER, S., and J. C. ECCLES (1930). 'Isometric muscle twitch.' *J. Physiol.* **69**, iii.

—, —— (1930). 'The isometric responses of mammalian muscles.' *J. Physiol.* **69**, 377.

58. CREED, R. S., and C. S. SHERRINGTON (1926). 'Observations on concurrent contraction of flexor muscles in the flexion reflex.' *Proc. Roy. Soc.* **100** B, 258.

59. CREED, R. S., and J. C. ECCLES (1928). 'The incidence of central inhibition on restricted fields of motor units.' *J. Physiol.* **66**, 109.

60. DAVIS, H. (1926). 'The conduction of the nerve impulse.' *Physiol. Rev.* **6**, 547.

61. DAVIS, L., and L. J. POLLOCK (1930). 'The peripheral pathway for painful sensations.' *Arch. Neurol. Psychiat. Chicago*, **24**, 883.

62. DENNY BROWN, D. (1928). 'On inhibition as a reflex accompaniment of the tendon-jerk and of other forms of active muscular response.' *Proc. Roy. Soc.* **103** B, 321.

63. —— (1929). 'On the nature of postural reflexes.' *Proc. Roy. Soc.* **104** B, 252.

64. —— (1929). 'The histological features of striped muscle in relation to its functional activity.' *Proc. Roy. Soc.* **104** B, 371.

65. —— Unpublished observations.

66. DENNY BROWN, D. E., and E. G. T. LIDDELL (1927). 'Observations on the motor twitch and on reflex inhibition of the tendon-jerk of M. supraspinatus.' *J. Physiol.* **63**, 70.

67. —, —— (1927). 'The stretch reflex as a spinal process.' *J. Physiol.* **63**, 144.

68. —, —— (1928). 'Extensor reflexes in the fore-limb.' *J. Physiol.* **65**, 305.

69. DENNY BROWN, D. E., and C. S. SHERRINGTON (1928). 'Subliminal fringe in spinal flexion.' *J. Physiol.* **66**, 175.

70. DOGIEL, A. S. (1906). 'Die Endigungen der sensiblen Nerven in den Augenmuskeln und deren Sehnen beim Menschen und den Säugetieren.' *Arch. mik. Anat.* **68**, 501.

71. DREYER, N. B., and C. S. SHERRINGTON (1918). 'Brevity, frequency of rhythm and amount of nervous reflex discharge, as indicated by reflex contraction.' *Proc. Roy. Soc.* **90** B, 270.

72. DUSSER DE BARENNE, J. G. (1911). 'Die electromotorischen Erscheinungen im Muskel bei der reziproken Innervation der quergestreiften Skelettmuskulatur.' *Zbl. Physiol.* **25**, 334.

73. DUSSER DE BARENNE and A. DE KLEYN (1931). 'On the reciprocal innervation of the eye-muscles.' *Acta. oto. laryng*, **16**, 97.

74. ECCLES, J. C. (1931). 'Studies on the flexor reflex. III. The central effects produced by an antidromic volley.' *Proc. Roy. Soc.* **107** B, 557.

75. ECCLES, J. C., and R. GRANIT (1929). 'Crossed extensor reflexes and their interaction.' *J. Physiol.* **67**, 97.

76. ——, —— Unpublished observations.

77. ECCLES, J. C., and C. S. SHERRINGTON (1930). 'Reflex summation in the ipselateral spinal flexion reflex.' *J. Physiol.* **69**, 1.

78. ——, —— (1930). 'Numbers and contraction-values of individual motor units examined in some muscles of the limb.' *Proc. Roy. Soc.* **106** B, 326.

79. ——, —— (1931). 'Studies on the flexor reflex. I. Latent period.' *Proc. Roy. Soc.* **107** B, 511.

80. ——, —— (1931). 'Studies on the flexor reflex. II. The reflex response evoked by two centripetal volleys.' *Proc. Roy. Soc.* **107** B, 535.

81. ——, —— (1931). 'Studies on the flexor reflex. IV. After-discharge.' *Proc. Roy. Soc.* **107** B, 586.

82. ——, —— (1931). 'Studies on the flexor reflex. V. General conclusions.' *Proc. Roy. Soc.* **107** B, 597.

83. ——, —— (1931). 'Studies on the flexor reflex. VI. Inhibition.' *Proc. Roy. Soc.* **109**, 91.

84. ERLANGER, J. (1927). 'The interpretation of the action potential in cutaneous and muscle nerves.' *Amer. J. Physiol.* **82**, 644.

85. ERLANGER, J., H. S. GASSER, and G. H. Bishop (1924). 'The compound nature of the action current of nerve as disclosed by the cathode ray oscillograph.' *Amer. J. Physiol.* **70**, 624; and subsequent papers in *Amer. J. Physiol.*

86. ——, ——, —— (1926). 'On conduction of the action potential wave through the dorsal root ganglion.' *Proc. Soc. Exp. Biol. N.Y.* **23**, 372.

87. ERLANGER, J., and H. S. GASSER (1930). 'The action potential in fibres of slow conduction in spinal roots and somatic nerves.' *Amer. J. Physiol.* **92**, 43.

88. FORBES, A. (1912). 'Reflex rhythm induced by concurrent excitation and inhibition.' *Proc. Roy. Soc.* **85** B, 289.

89. —— (1922). 'The interpretation of spinal reflexes in terms of present knowledge of nerve conduction.' *Physiol. Rev.* **2**, 361.

90. FORBES, A., and A. GREGG (1915). 'Electrical studies in mammalian reflexes. I. The flexion reflex.' *Amer. J. Physiol.* **37**, 118.

91. FORBES, A., C. J. CAMPBELL, and H. B. WILLIAMS (1924). 'Electrical records of afferent nerve impulses from muscular receptors.' *Amer. J. Physiol.* **69**, 283.

92. FORBES, A., and McK. CATTELL (1924). 'Electrical studies in

mammalian reflexes. IV. The crossed extension reflex.' *Amer. J. Physiol.* **70**, 140.
93. FORBES, A., A. QUERIDO, L. R. WHITAKER, and L. M. HURXTHAL (1928). 'Electrical studies in mammalian reflexes. V. The flexion reflex in response to two stimuli as recorded from the motor-nerve.' *Amer. J. Physiol.* **85**, 432.
94. FORBES, A., H. DAVIS, and E. LAMBERT (1930). 'The conflict between excitatory and inhibitory effects in a spinal centre.' *Amer. J. Physiol.* **95**, 142.
95. FULTON, J. F. (1926). *Muscular contraction and the reflex control of movement.* Baltimore and London.
96. —— (1930). *Selected readings from the history of physiology.* Baltimore.
97. FULTON, J. F., and E. G. T. LIDDELL (1925). 'Observations on ipselateral contraction and "inhibitory" rhythm.' *Proc. Roy. Soc.* **98** B, 214.
98. FULTON, J. F., and J. PI-SUÑER (1927). 'A note concerning the probable function of various afferent end-organs in skeletal muscle.' *Amer. J. Physiol.* **83**, 554.
99. FULTON, J. F., E. G. T. LIDDELL, and D. McK. RIOCH (1930). 'The influence of experimental lesions of the spinal cord under the knee-jerk.' *Brain*, **53**, 311.
100. ——, ——, —— (1930). 'The influence of unilateral destruction of the vestibular nuclei upon posture and the knee-jerk.' *Brain*, **53**, 327.
101. FULTON, J. F., and A. D. KELLER (1932). *The Babinski reflex in the monkey, baboon, and chimpanzee.* Baltimore.

102. GASSER, H. S., and J. ERLANGER (1925). 'The nature of conduction of an impulse in the relatively refractory period.' *Amer. J. Physiol.* **73**, 613.
103. ——, ——- (1930). 'The ending of the axon action potential, and its relation to other events in nerve activity.' *Amer. J. Physiol.* **94**, 247.
104. GERARD, R. W., and A. FORBES (1928). ' "Fatigue" of the flexion reflex.' *Amer. J. Physiol.* **86**, 186.

105. HERRICK, C. J. (1924). *Neurological foundations of animal behaviour.* New York.
106. HILL, A. V. (1929). 'The heat-production and recovery of crustacean nerve.' *Proc. Roy. Soc.* **105** B, 153.
107. HINSEY, J. C. (1927). 'Some observations on the innervation of skeletal muscle of the cat.' *J. Comp. Neurol.* **44**, 87.
108. HOLMES, GORDON M. (1915). 'The pathology of acute spinal injuries.' Goulstonian Lectures. *Brit. Med. J.* ii. 769.
109. HUBER, G. C., and L. M. A. DE WITT (1900). 'A contribution on

the nerve terminations in neurotendinous end-organs.' *J. Comp. Neurol.* **10**, 159.

110. INGBERT, C. (1903). 'An enumeration of the medullated nerve-fibres in the dorsal roots of the spinal nerves of man.' *J. Comp. Neurol.* **13**, 53; and 'On the density of the cutaneous innervation in man.' *Ibid.* **53**, 209.

111. JOLLY, W. A. (1911). 'On the time relations of the knee-jerk and simple reflexes.' *Quart. J. Exp. Physiol.* **4**, 67.

112. DE KLEYN, A. (1923). 'Experimental physiology of the labyrinth.' *J. Laryng. Lond.* **38**, 645.
113. DE KLEYN, A., and C. VERSTEEGH (1927). 'Some remarks upon the present position of the physiology of the labyrinth.' *J. Laryng. Lond.* **42**, 649.

114. LABHART, F. (1929). 'Fortgesetzte Untersuchungen über den Einfluss des Nervus sympathicus auf die Ermüdung des quergestreiften Muskels.' *Z. Biol.* **89**, 217 (from the laboratory of Prof. L. Asher).
115. LAPICQUE, L. (1925). 'Sur la théorie de l'addition latente.' *Ann. physiol. physicochem. biol.* **1**, 133.
116. LIDDELL, E. G. T., and C. S. SHERRINGTON (1923). 'Stimulus rhythm in reflex tetanic contraction.' *Proc. Roy. Soc.* **95 B**, 142.
117. ——, —— (1923). 'A comparison between certain features of the spinal flexor reflex and of the decerebrate extensor reflex respectively.' *Proc. Roy. Soc.* **95 B**, 299.
118. ——, —— (1923). 'Recruitment type of reflexes.' *Proc. Roy. Soc.* **95 B**, 407.
119. ——, —— (1924). 'Reflexes in response to stretch (myotatic reflexes).' *Proc. Roy. Soc.* **96 B**, 212.
120. ——, —— (1925). 'Further observations on myotatic reflexes.' *Proc. Roy. Soc.* **97 B**, 267.
121. ——, —— (1925). 'Recruitment and some other features of reflex inhibition.' *Proc. Roy. Soc.* **97 B**, 488.
122. LIDDELL, E. G. T., and J. M. D. OLMSTED (1929). 'The effect of the responses of the soleus muscle of an alcohol block on the sciatic nerve.' *J. Physiol.* **67**, 33.
123. LILLIE, R. S. (1922). 'Transmission of physiological influence in protoplasmic systems, especially nerve.' *Physiol. Rev.* **2**, 1.
124. LUCAS, K. (1910). 'Quantitative researches on the summation of inadequate stimuli in muscle and nerve, with observations on the time-factor in electric stimulation.' *J. Physiol.* **39**, 461.
125. —— (1917). *The conduction of the nervous impulse.* London.

204   REFERENCES

126. McCouch, G. P., A. Forbes, and L. H. Rice (1928). 'Afferent impulses from muscular receptors.' *Amer. J. Physiol.* **84**, 1.
127. Magnus, R. (1924). *Körperstellung.* Berlin.
128. —— (1926). 'Some results of studies in the physiology of posture.' Cameron Prize Lectures. *Lancet. Lond.* **2**, 211, 531, 585.
129. Maibach, C. (1928). 'Untersuchungen zur Frage des Einflusses des Sympathikus auf die Ermüdung der quergestreiften Muskulatur.' *Z. Biol.* **88**, 207 (from the laboratory of Prof. L. Asher).
130. Mathews, B. H. C. (1928). 'A new electrical recording system for physiological work.' *J. Physiol.* **65**, 225.
131. —— (1931). 'The response of a single end organ.' *J. Physiol.* **71**, 64.
132. —— (1931). 'The response of a muscle-spindle during active contraction of a muscle.' *J. Physiol.* **72**, 153.

133. Nevin, S. (1930). 'Degeneration change after unilateral lumbar sympathectomy, with general observations on the nerve-fibre constitution of peripheral nerves and nerve-roots.' *Quart. J. Exp. Physiol.* **20**, 281.

134. Orbeli, L. A. (1924). Pavlov Jubilee Volume, Leningrad. For account in English see 'The autonomic nervous system', by A. Kuntz, 1929.
135. Owen, A. G. W., and C. S. Sherrington (1911). 'Observations on strychnine reversal.' *J. Physiol.* **43**, 232.

136. Penfield, W. G. (1921). 'The Golgi apparatus and its relationship to Holgren's trophospongium in nerve-cells. Comparison during retispersion.' *Anat. Rec.* **22**, 57.
137. Philippson, M. (1905). 'L'autonomie et la centralisation dans le système nerveux des animaux.' *Trav. Lab. Inst. Physiol. Brux.* **7**, ii. 1.
138. Phillips, G. (1931). 'On posture and postural reflex action: the effect of unilateral lumbar sympathetic chain observation.' *Brain*, **54**, 320.
139. —— (1932). *In the press.*
140. Pi-Suñer, J., and J. F. Fulton (1929). 'The influence of the proprioceptive system upon the crossed extensor reflex.' *Amer. J. Physiol.* **88**, 453.
141. Pollock, L. J., and L. Davis (1930). 'Reflex activities of a decerebrate animal.' *J. Comp. Neurol.* **50**, 377.
142. ——, —— (1931). 'The effect of deafferentation on decerebrate rigidity.' *Amer. J. Physiol.* **98**, 47.
143. Pritchard, E. A. B. (1926). 'Die Stützreaktion.' *Pfluegers Arch.* **214**, 148.

144. QUERIDO, A. (1924). 'The function of the peripheral neurones in the conduction of impulses in the sympathetic nervous system.' *Amer. J. Physiol.* **70**, 29.

145. RADEMAKER, G. G. J. (1931). *Das Stehen.* Berlin.
146. RANSON, S. W. (1929). 'The parasympathetic control of muscle tonus.' *Arch. Neurol. Psychiat. Chicago*, **22**, 265.
147. RIDDOCH, G. (1917). 'The reflex functions of the completely divided spinal cord in man, compared with those associated with less severe lesions.' *Brain*, **40**, 264.
148. ROAF, H. E., and C. S. SHERRINGTON (1910). 'Further remarks on the spinal mammalian preparation.' *Quart. J. Exp. Physiol.* **3**, 209.
149. RUFFINI, A. (1898). 'On the minute anatomy of the neuromuscular spindles of the cat and on their physiological significance.' *J. Physiol.* **23**, 190.

150. SAMOJLOFF, A., and M. KISSELEFF (1927). 'Zur Charakteristik der zentralen Hemmungsprozesse.' *Pfluegers Arch.* **215**, 699.
151. SCHAFER, E. A. (1878). 'Observations on the nervous system of *Aurelia aurita*.' *Phil. Trans.* **169**, 563.
152. SCHAFER, E. A., SHARPEY—, and H. M. CARLETON (1929). *The essentials of histology.* London.
153. SCHOEN, R. (1926). 'Die Stützreaktion.' *Pfluegers Arch.* **214**, 21.
154. SHERRINGTON, C. S. (1892). 'Notes on the arrangement of some motor-fibres in the lumbo-sacral plexus.' *J. Physiol.* **13**, 621.
155. —— (1893). 'Note on the knee-jerk and the correlation of action of antagonistic muscles.' *Proc. Roy. Soc.* **52**, 556.
156. —— (1893). 'Further experimental note on the correlation of action of antagonistic muscles.' *Proc. Roy. Soc.* **53**, 407.
157. —— (1894). 'Experimental note on two movements of the eye.' *J. Physiol.* **17**, 27.
158. —— (1894). 'On the anatomical constitution of nerves of skeletal muscles; with remarks on recurrent fibres in the ventral spinal nerve-root.' *J. Physiol.* **17**, 211.
159. —— (1898). 'Decerebrate rigidity, and reflex co-ordination of movements.' *J. Physiol.* **22**, 319.
160. —— (1898). 'Experiments in examination of the peripheral distribution of the fibres of the posterior roots of some spinal nerves, Part II.' Croonian Lecture, 1897. *Philos. Trans.* **190**, 45.
161. —— (1900). 'On the innervation of antagonistic muscles. Sixth note.' *Proc. Roy. Soc.* **66**, 66.
162. —— (1900). Special articles by, in Schafer's *Text-book of Physiology*, vol. ii. Edinburgh.
163. —— (1903). 'Qualitative difference of spinal reflex corresponding

206 REFERENCES

with qualitative difference of cutaneous stimulus.' *J. Physiol.* **30**, 39.

164. SHERRINGTON, C. S. (1904). 'Correlation of reflexes and the principle of the common path.' *Rep. Brit. Ass.* 1904, 728.

165. —— (1905). 'On reciprocal innervation of antagonistic muscles. Seventh note.' *Proc. Roy. Soc.* **76**, 160.

166. —— (1905). 'On reciprocal innervation of antagonistic muscles. Eighth note.' *Proc. Roy. Soc.* **76**, 269.

167. —— (1906). 'Observations on the scratch reflex in the spinal dog.' *J. Physiol.* **34**, 1.

168. —— (1906). *The integrative action of the nervous system.* New Haven and London.

169. —— (1906). 'On innervation of antagonistic muscles. Ninth note. Successive spinal induction.' *Proc. Roy. Soc.* **77** B, 478.

170. —— (1907). 'On reciprocal innervation of antagonistic muscles. Tenth note.' *Proc. Roy. Soc.* **79** B, 337.

171. —— (1908). 'Some comparisons between reflex inhibition and reflex excitation.' *Quart. J. Exp. Physiol.* **1**, 67.

172. —— (1908). 'On reciprocal innervation of antagonistic muscles. Eleventh note. Further observations on successive induction.' *Proc. Roy. Soc.* **80** B, 53.

173. —— (1908). 'On reciprocal innervation of antagonistic muscles. Twelfth note. Proprioceptive reflexes.' *Proc. Roy. Soc.* **80** B, 552.

174. —— (1908). 'On reciprocal innervation of antagonistic muscles. Thirteenth note. On the antagonism between reflex inhibition and reflex excitation.' *Proc. Roy. Soc.* **80** B, 565.

175. —— (1909). 'Reciprocal innervation of antagonistic muscles. Fourteenth note. On double reciprocal innervation.' *Proc. Roy. Soc.* **81** B, 249.

176. —— (1909). 'A mammalian spinal preparation.' *J. Physiol.* **38**, 375.

177. —— (1909). 'On plastic tonus and proprioceptive reflexes.' *Quart. J. Exp. Physiol.* **2**, 109.

178. —— (1910). 'Flexion reflex of the limb, crossed extension reflex, and reflex stepping and standing.' *J. Physiol.* **40**, 28.

179. —— (1913). 'Reciprocal innervation of symmetrical muscles.' *Proc. Roy. Soc.* **86** B, 219.

180. —— (1913). 'Nervous rhythm arising from rivalry of antagonistic reflexes: reflex stepping as outcome of double reciprocal innervation.' *Proc. Roy. Soc.* **86** B, 233.

181. —— (1913). 'Reflex inhibition as a factor in the co-ordination of movements and postures.' *Quart. J. Exp. Physiol.* **6**, 251.

182. —— (1915). 'Postural activity of muscle and nerve.' *Brain*, **38**, 191.

183. —— (1917). 'Reflexes elicitable in the cat from pinna, vibrissae, and jaws.' *J. Physiol.* **51**, 404.

184. SHERRINGTON, C. S. (1919). 'Note on the history of the word "tonus" as a physiological term.' Contributions to medical and biological research, dedicated to Sir William Osler. Vol. 1, p. 261. New York.

185. —— (1921). 'Break-shock reflexes and "supramaximal" contraction-response of mammalian nerve-muscle to single shock stimuli.' *Proc. Roy. Soc.* **92** B, 245.

186. —— (1921). 'Sur la production d'influx nerveux dans l'arc nerveux réflexe.' *Arch. int. Physiol.* **18**, 620.

187. —— (1924). 'Problems of muscular receptivity.' *Nature*, **113**, 732, 892, and 924.

188. —— (1925). 'Remarks on some aspects of reflex inhibition.' *Proc. Roy. Soc.* **97** B, 519.

189. —— (1926). 'Addition latente and recruitment in reflex contraction and inhibition,' from *Livre à Charles Richet*. Paris.

190. —— (1929).—'Some functional problems attaching to convergence.' Ferrier Lecture. *Proc. Roy. Soc.* **105** B, 332.

191. —— (1931). 'Quantitative management of contraction in lowest level co-ordination.' Hughlings Jackson Lecture. *Brain*, **54**, 1.

192. SHERRINGTON, C. S., and S. C. M. SOWTON (1911). 'Chloroform and reversal of reflex effect.' *J. Physiol.* **42**, 383.

193. ——, —— (1911). 'Reversal of the reflex effect of an afferent nerve by altering the character of the electrical stimulus applied.' *Proc. Roy. Soc.* **83** B, 435.

194. ——, —— (1911). 'On reflex inhibition of the knee flexor.' *Proc. Roy. Soc.* **84** B, 201.

195. ——, —— (1911). *Reflex rebound*. Liverpool. (Cited also by Forbes, Davis, and Lambert, cf. 94.)

196. ——, —— (1915). 'Observations on reflex responses to single break-shocks.' *J. Physiol.* **49**, 331.

197. SPIEGEL, E. A. (1927). 'Der Tonus der Skelettmuskulatur.' *Monogr. a. d. Gesamtgeb. d. Neurol. u. Psychol.* 51.

198. TIEGS, O. W. (1927). 'A critical review of the evidence on which is based the theory of discontinuous synapses in the spinal cord.' *Aust. J. Exp. Biol. Med. Sci.* **4**, 193.

199. —— (1931). 'A study of the neurofibril structure of the nerve-cell.' *J. Comp. Neurol.* **52**, 189.

200. TOWER, S. S. (1931). 'A search for trophic influence of posterior spinal roots on skeletal muscle, with a note on the nerve-fibres found in the proximal stumps of the roots after excision of the root ganglia.' *Brain*, **54**, 99.

201. TOZER, F. M., and C. S. SHERRINGTON (1910). 'Receptors and afferents of the third, fourth, and sixth cranial nerves.' *Proc. Roy. Soc.* **82** B, 450.

202. VERWORN, M. (1900). 'Zur Physiologie der nervösen Hemmungserscheinungen.' *Arch. Physiol.* Suppl. vol., 105.

203. VIETS, H. (1920). 'Relation of the form of the knee-jerk and patellar clonus to muscle tonus.' *Brain*, **43**, 269.
204. VON BRÜCKE, E. T. (1922). 'Zur Theorie der intrazentralen Hemmungen.' *Z. Biol.* **77**, 29.
205. VON BRÜCKE, E. T., C. L. HOU, and E. KRANNICH (1931). 'Rebound und intrazentraler Wettstreit zwischen hemmenden und erregenden Impulsen.' *Pfluegers Arch.* **227**, 733.

206. WARRINGTON, W. B. (1904). 'Note on the ultimate fate of ventral cornual cells after section of a number of posterior roots.' *J. Physiol.* **30**, 503.
207. WEISS, G., and A. DUTIL (1896). 'Recherches sur le fuseau neuro-musculaire.' *Arch. de Physiol.* **28**, 368.
208. HOFF, E. C. (1932). 'Degeneration of the *boutons terminaux* in the spinal cord.' *J. Physiol.* **74**, 4 P.
209. McCOUCH, G. P. (1924). 'The relation of the pyramidal tract to spinal shock.' *Amer. J. Physiol.* **71**, 137.

REFERENCES TO THE ANNOTATIONS

210. BARRON, D. H. and MATTHEWS, B. H. C. (1938) The interpretation of potential changes in the spinal cord. *J. Physiol.* **92**, 276.
211. BODIAN, D. (1949) In *Poliomyelitis*, papers presented at the first International poliomyelitis Conference, Philadelphia, Lippincott, p. 62.
212. BOYD, I. A. and DAVEY, M. R. (1968) *Composition of peripheral nerves.* Livingstone, Edinburgh, and London.
213. BROOKS, C. McC. and FUORTES, M. G. F. (1952) Electrical correlates of the spinal flexor reflex. *Brain* **75**, 91.
214. ECCLES, J. C. (1964) *The physiology of synapses.* Springer Verlag, Berlin, Göttingen, Heidelberg.
215. EDISEN, A. E. U. (1956) Excitation and inhibition of spinal motoneurons. *Am. J. Physiol.* **184**, 223.
216. —— (1967) Primary afferent fibres of contralateral origin in the lower spinal cord of the cat. *Expl Neurol.* **18**, 38.
217. ERLANGER, J. and GASSER, H. S. (1968) *Electrical signs of nervous activity*, 2nd edn. U. Penna Press, Philadelphia.
218. FRANK, K. (1959) Basic mechanisms of synaptic transmission in the nervous system. *I.R.E. Trans. med. Electron.* **ME6**, 85.
219. FRANK, K. and FUORTES, M. G. F. (1957) Presynaptic and postsynaptic inhibition of monosynaptic reflexes. *Fedn Proc. Fedn Am. Socs exp. Biol.* **16**, 39.
220. GASSER, H. S. (1935) Changes in nerve-potentials produced by rapidly repeated stimuli and their relation to the responsiveness of nerve to stimulation. *Am. J. Physiol.* **111**, 35.

221. GASSER, H. S. (1950) Unmedullated fibres originating in dorsal root ganglia. *J. gen. Physiol.* **33**, 651.

222. —— (1955) Properties of unmedullated fibres on the two sides of the ganglion. *J. gen. Physiol.* **38**, 709.

223. —— (1960) Effect of the method of leading on the recording of the nerve fibre spectrum. *J. gen. Physiol.* **43**, 927.

224. GASSER, H. S. and GRAHAM, H. T. (1933) Potentials produced in the spinal cord by stimulation of dorsal roots. *Am. J. Physiol.* **103**, 303.

225. GRANIT, R. (Ed.) (1966) *Nobel Symposium, I, Muscular afferents and motor control.* Almqvist and Wicksel, Stockholm.

226. HARTLINE, H. K., MARK, R. F., and STEINER, J. (1956) Inhibition in the eye of *Limulus. J. gen. Physiol.* **39**, 651.

227. HUGHES, J. and GASSER, H. S. (1934) Some properties of the cord potentials evoked by a single afferent volley. *Am. J. Physiol.* **108**, 295.

228. —— —— (1934) The response of the cord to two afferent volleys. *Am. J. Physiol.* **108**, 307.

229. HUNT, C. C. (1955) Monosynaptic reflex response of spinal motoneurones to graded afferent stimulation. *J. gen. Physiol.* **38**, 813.

230. LAPORTE, Y. and LLOYD, D. P. C. (1952) Nature and significance of the reflex connections established by large afferent fibres of muscular origin. *Am. J. Physiol.* **169**, 609.

231. LLOYD, D. P. C. (1941) A direct inhibitory action of dromically conducted impulses. *J. Neurophysiol.* **4**, 184.

232. —— (1941) The spinal mechanism of the pyramidal system in cats. *J. Neurophysiol.* **4**, 435.

233. —— (1943) The interaction of antidromic and orthodromic volleys in a segmental spinal motor nucleus. *J. Neurophysiol.* **6**, 143.

234. —— (1943) Neuron patterns controlling transmission of ipsilateral hind limb reflexes in cat. *J. Neurophysiol.* **6**, 293.

235. —— (1943) Conduction and synaptic transmission of reflex response to stretch in spinal cats. *J. Neurophysiol.* **6**, 317.

236. —— (1944) Functional organization of the spinal cord. *Physiol. Rev.* **44**, 1.

237. —— (1945) On the relation between discharge zone and subliminal fringe in a motoneurone pool supplied by a homogenious presynaptic pathway. *Yale J. Biol. Med.* **18**, 117.

238. —— (1951) After-currents, after-potentials, excitability and ventral root electrotonus in spinal motoneurones. *J. gen. Physiol.* **35**, 289.

239. —— (1955) Principles of nervous activity. In *Textbook of physiology,* 17th edn. Saunders, Philadelphia.

240. —— (1957). Input–output relation in a flexor reflex. *J. gen. Physiol.* **41**, 297.

241. LLOYD, D. P. C. (1957) Temporal summation in rhythmically active monosynaptic reflex pathways. *J. gen. Physiol.* **40**, 427.

242. —— (1959) The discrete and the diffuse in nervous action. James Arthur lecture, The American Museum of Natural History.

243. —— (1959) Temperature and dendritic response of spinal neurons. *Proc. natn. Acad. Sci. U.S.A.* **45**, 589.

244. —— (1960) Spinal mechanisms in somatic activities. *Handbook of physiology-neurophysiology II*, Chap. 36, p. 929.

245. —— (1970) Early recovery of antidromic conduction through dendrites of spinal neurones in the normal, anoxic and post anoxic states. *Proc. natn. Acad. Sci. U.S.A.* **66**, 622.

246. —— (1970) Excitatory postsynaptic potential and monosynaptic reflex discharge of spinal motoneurones during anoxic insult. *Proc. natn. Acad. Sci. U.S.A.* **66**, 626.

247. —— (1970) Action in primary afferent fibers in the spinal cord. *Int. J. Neurosci.* **1**, 1.

248. —— and CHANG, H-T. (1948) Afferent fibers in motor nerves. *J. Neurophysiol.* **11**, 199.

249. —— and MCINTYRE, A. K. (1950) Dorsal column conduction of Group I afferent impulses and their relay through Clarke's column. *J. Neurophysiol.* **13**, 39.

250. —— and WILSON, V. J. (1959) Functional organization in the terminal segments of the spinal cord with a consideration of excitatory and inhibitory latencies in monosynaptic reflex systems. *J. gen. Physiol.* **42**, 1219.

251. LORENTE DE NÓ, R. (1947) A study of nerve physiology. *Stud. Rockefeller Inst. med. Res.* **131, 132**, 496, 548.

252. —— (1953) Conduction of impulses in the neurones of the oculomotor nucleus. In *The spinal cord, A Ciba Foundation Symposium*, p. 132.

253. MATTHEWS, P. B. C. (1962) The differentiation of two types of fusimotor fibre by their effects of the dynamic response of muscle spindle primary endings. *Q. Jl. exp. Physiol.* **47**, 324.

254. MCINTYRE, A. K. (1965) Some applications of input–output technique. In *Studies in physiology.* Springer-Verlag, Berlin, Heidelberg, New York.

255. —— MARK, R. F. and STEINER, J. (1956) Multiple firing at central synapses. *Nature, Lond.* **178**, 302.

256. PERL, E. R. (1957) Crossed reflexes of cutaneous origin. *Am. J. Physiol.* **188**, 609.

257. —— (1958) Crossed reflex effects evoked by activity in myelinated afferent fibres of muscle. *J. Neurophysiol.* **21**, 101.

258. —— (1959) Effects of muscle stretch on excitability of contralateral motoneurones. *J. Physiol.* **145**, 193.

259. RENSHAW, B. (1941) Influence of the discharge of motoneurones upon excitation of neighbouring motoneurones. *J. Neurophysiol.* **4**, 167.

260. RENSHAW, B. (1942) Effects of presynaptic volleys on spread of impulses over the soma of the motoneurone. *J. Neurophysiol.* **5**, 235.

261. RUSHTON, W. A. H. (1937) Initiation of the propogated disturbance. *Proc. R. Soc.* **B124**, 201.

262. SCHÄFER, E. A. (1899) Some results of partial transverse section of the spinal cord. *J. Physiol.* **24**, XXXII.

263. SCHEIBEL, M. E. and SCHEIBEL, A. B. (1969) Terminal patterns in cat spinal cord. III Primary afferent collaterals. *Brain Res.* **13**, 417.

264. SVAETICHIN, G. (1951). Electrophysiological investigations on single ganglion cells. *Acta physiol scand.* **24**, Suppl. 86, 1.

265. TOENNIES, J. F. (1938) Reflex discharge from the spinal cord over the dorsal roots. *J. Neurophysiol.* **1**, 378.

266. WILSON, V. J. (1959) Recurrent facilitation of spinal reflexes. *J. gen. Physiol.* **42**, 703.

INDEX